Restore Your Life!

Powerful Life Strategies To Navigate Menopause

Kelly Nolan, BSc. Pharm.
Women's Health Expert and Owner of Avita Integrative Health

Published by Prominence Publishing.

www.prominencepublishing.com

The author can be reached as follows:

Avita Integrative Health
Email: kelly@avitaintegrativehealth.ca
Website: hormonetesting.ca
Phone: 416-884-8444

Restore Your Life/Kelly Nolan. -- 1st ed.

ISBN: 978-1-990830-08-2

Dedication

I would like to dedicate this book with gratitude to my "inner strength" and "utmost courage" to face life's challenges. In the middle of writing this book I found myself on a very different, unexpected pathway. A pathway that created another layer of respect and understanding for all women face through their never-ending responsibilities & commitment to others. Sharing my life experiences with authenticity greatly influenced the content of this book and my continued passion to teach women the importance of self-care... this is my story.

Dear Jennifer,
Thank you for trusting in my expertise! May you find the tools & resources in this book to successfully support & embrace your menopause journey.
Please pay it forward to someone in your community struggling for answers. ENJOY!
Kelly

Note from the Author

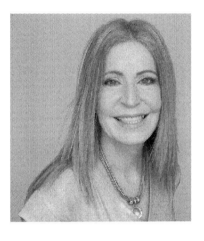

As a women's health expert, once I discovered the key to solving my own worst menopause symptoms, I realized I could not keep this secret to myself. My mission was very clear... I needed to reach a broad audience of women to educate and support their journey to minimize their feelings of frustration, disappointment and low self-esteem. To let them know there are answers!

After discovering the blueprint to moving past my worst menopausal symptoms, I knew my obligation was to share my secret with women struggling with menopause. I need women to know there are solutions. I never want them to just give up and accept their symptoms as a part of aging!

By sharing my expertise with authenticity and compassion, I have mentored their passage through menopause with real, science-based solutions to take control back and have the body they want!

Kelly Nolan, BSc. Pharm

Acknowledgements

To my clients: You have supported my vision and trusted in my knowledge and expertise over the years. Truly believing, as I do, in the value of Integrative Medicine, its strength in the treatment and prevention of disease, and support of our whole-body health.

To my longest standing client, Anne G, who at 70 is still religious with the herbs to support her health with little to no medication: We have laughed together and at times have come close to tears in sharing our life experiences.

To one of my favourite clients, Sue W, who encouraged me to be transparent and real without fear of judgement. To remove all barriers and confide in women to build trusting relationships. To share life experiences in the hopes that, as women, we can learn from each other.

To all the women who embraced my expertise and continue to do so with the strong belief that menopause is a chapter of life to celebrate. That we never have to give up. We can take control back and have the life we so desire! The last chapter!

What People Are Saying...

Angela Kafadar, Owner, VideoPowerup:

Being through menopause at a young age, I was confused and miserable. There were so many things I went through that I just thought were normal and there was nothing I could have done! I wish (if not for the night sweats, for the pure sake of my sex life!) I would have read this sooner. I connected with many of the stories and had so many "Aha" moments. The book is not only empowering but could be life changing as a woman who went through menopause in her 40's.

Mary Anne Cairns, Founder, Wellpoint Wellness Group:

Kelly Nolan is a dedicated Health Professional who will inspire, educate, and guide women through every aspect of the menopause experience. Learn more about the health issues that arise with menopause and which strategies and solutions could be helpful in navigating this transition. Many women will relate to the stories in this interactive book. Menopause is a natural part of aging; this excellent book will help women to embrace this stage of their life with confidence and clarity!

Kelly Erais, Owner & CEO, Whole Body Fitness:

Kelly, I have had the utmost pleasure to go through your book. What a great resource with so much important info! I love your approach from a whole health perspective, looking at much more than just the physical but also the mental health challenges during menopause, as well; a factor I think is still somehow so often overlooked. I'd be thrilled to buy a few copies for my library and clients I know are struggling through menopause. My favourite part − "Hot flashes, a sudden volcanic eruption of body heat from your chest, neck, and face!"

Lori McCrae, CMO and Owner, NexGEN Marketing Group:

"Before I read Kelly's book, I felt like I was alone on my menopause journey. Reading this book is like having a friend through menopause. Kelly provides an expert's perspective on how to live your best life through the menopause years. With this book, I now have the tools to get my health on track and live the life I so desire."

Table of Contents

UNDERSTANDING MY MENOPAUSE JOURNEY

My 'WHY'

Menopause is part of aging, but you don't have to just accept feeling confused, insecure, and not like yourself. You can feel like an informed participant in your own health and wellbeing. You can be the architect of your own plan.

You may be wondering about the person who has put this resource together for you, and what brought me to the point where I had to commit my knowledge, personal experience, and passion to writing and finding a way to share my expertise with other women. After discovering the blueprint to moving past the worst menopausal symptoms I knew my obligation was to share the secret with women struggling with menopause. I needed women to know there are solutions. I never wanted them to just give up and accept their symptoms as a part of aging!

This book is the result of my own successful journey, and my work with hundreds of women over the past 25 years. The greatest affirmation of my work is that so many of my clients have become trusting friends. We have grown and learned from each other along the way.

Knowing that people receive and respond to information in different ways, I have developed this resource as a big picture to be as accessible as possible. It's a step-by-step guide that sets a foundation of knowledge as our starting point, providing background details in both scientific and plain language terms. I want to inform, not overwhelm you.

I'm going to introduce you to some people you can identify with, or who may remind you of someone you know. I've also made this book interactive. I want you to get out your pencil and make notes and highlight sections that are meaningful.

My goal is that, as you get to know the facts, you get to know yourself. The power of information is knowledge, and knowledge means choice. And choice is gaining control back into our day-to-day lives.

My Start

I grew up in a small town in Northern Ontario in a 'normal' middle-class family with my parents and older sister. It seems unbelievable to look back on it now, but nothing in my life ever went wrong! Things unfolded for me as expected, and I went along with the flow, secure that I was following a plan.

Despite this, I do recognize I grew up with very low self-esteem which carried forward into adulthood until I met my second husband.

I'm a 'science type' and always knew I wanted to work in a field that involves helping people, but I wasn't sure what. I tried a physiotherapy placement in high school, but that wasn't a fit. My parents said they would pay for school if I did the work, so I attended the University of British Columbia (UBC). I took one year of science before I found my place and graduated as a pharmacist in 1987. Everything was going to plan.

However, just prior to graduating, the first life-altering event occurred in my life in January 1987. I was in a near-fatal car accident. I was in the passenger seat when the car ended up wrapped around a hydro pole. It took over 45 minutes and the jaws of life to remove me from the wreckage. My pelvis was broken in four places as well as my left ankle. I was extremely lucky to be alive. The police officer later told my sister he was very scared to look in the car.

After spending a month in the hospital, I went back to school in a wheelchair, while I learned how to walk again. It took extreme courage to overcome my physical challenges. It was extremely painful, but I was told I would have to be patient and heal. I was fearful and anxious knowing that my life could have easily ended that fateful night.

I could have postponed my last semester and returned to school in September, but I decided to push through and graduate with my class.

No one gave me a pass; I had to finish every test, every exam, and every internship.

It was the first time I became aware of my inner strength of character and determination to succeed. I never gave up, and I graduated! Then I returned to my hometown, and on July 25th, 1987, I walked down the aisle and married my first husband. We moved to Toronto, and I continued my career as a pharmacist, believing that medication would save the world!

Fast forward to 1997, after my third child was born, when I met and befriended Maria, a breast cancer survivor. Maria turned my head 180 degrees and taught me the benefits of utilizing pharmaceutical-grade herbal supplements and detoxification to support my health and the health of my children. At first, I just listened politely when she shared what she knew. I was a pharmacist, after all. What could she teach me…? I listened politely, but I thought it was all a bit of hocus pocus.

I started to learn more about the history and practice of Integrative Medicine, and how it places the individual at the centre of care, rather than the symptom or disease. A holistic medical approach takes into account the lifestyle habits of a patient and treats them as a whole person, not an isolated issue or complaint. The Integrative Practitioner works to treat the whole person rather than just the disease. The mind, body, and soul of a patient are taken into consideration to promote healing and well-being. It puts the patient in a more powerful position than in conventional medicine, able to understand recommendations and to make choices about their care. It also connects other choices people make to what they're feeling and experiencing, meaning changes in diet, exercise, responses to stress, habits, and much more can be connected to the immediate complaint or concern.

I had invested years in university and had 10 years' experience as a professional pharmacist. However this was the beginning of my transition to following a new pathway of learning and embracing Integrative Medicine. As I look back, I truly understand the Law of Attraction and why the universe brought Maria into my world! While

Maria is no longer with us, I think of her often and thank her dearly for giving me the gift of learning, and the opportunity for choice.

I learned more about integrative health. It is an individualized, client-centred model of promoting optimal health and wellness, combining a whole person approach with evidence-based strategies to reduce disease risk by turning around lifestyle behaviours.

It doesn't just treat disease,
but actively works to reduce disease in the first place.

Let me give you an example. Rather than recommending you take a prescription (such as Zantac or Pepcid) every day for heartburn, Integrative Medicine would look at multiple possible contributors or aggravators. How much dairy do you consume? How much caffeine are you consuming? Do you eat fatty foods? What's your stress level? How do you manage stress? Do you struggle with bloating and/or constipation?

At work I was dispensing medications to 40-year-olds that I used to dispense to 70-year-olds. The more I learned about Integrative Medicine the more excited I was. I recognized there was another way. And it made sense. I was learning at a time when my mind was open. And I was starting to think about moving away from the pharmaceutical industry.

I could still help people, but in a different way and, I believed, a better way.

Unfortunately, at that time, I was in denial that my marriage was in ruins after four children and 25 years. This was my second life-altering event. I had to face reality that my marriage was over. This was never part of the plan. In the beginning, it felt like a very catastrophic event in my life and the lives of my children. Fearful of being alone, I had to execute a very careful exit strategy.

I carried this burden for a long time, keeping it from family and clients, feeling like a failure. One day, a very good client asked why I wasn't wearing my wedding rings, and we both shared our stories. This was a turning point in my career. Because of Sue, I started to open my heart and soul to my clients, sharing my life experiences. I became 'real and relatable,' always speaking from my heart. This was scary at first, but the rewards were real, for both me and my clients in building strong and trusting relationships.

In 2012, my husband and I divorced. When my clients would give me their condolences, I would tell them that it was time for me to go on to the next chapter of my life, as I also realized that this marriage was holding back the success of my business. My perception of my new life became positive, and I began to approach this chapter with confidence. I had a plan again.

After divorce, I devoted myself to my work and my children, determined to be successful on my own. I also began to put self-care first again, lost 30 pounds, and re-entered the world with renewed self-esteem and a fresh self-image.

Flash forward to 2016 and I married my second husband on a private beach in Bahamas. Together we dreamed of building a life in Bahamas as it had become our second home, the place where we fell in love.

After my brief encounter with breast cancer in 2021, a gift to change my life, I started to take inventory of what wasn't working in my life and feeling very grateful for what was. Unfortunately, I faced the death of yet another marriage. I decided it was time to set healthy boundaries as I listened to my inner voice and celebrated my good fortune of full recovery, setting goals for the next chapter of my life. Within six months, I had lost a breast and a marriage. Accepting my aloneness, I soon began to enjoy a structured day full of solitude, peace, my work, and the company of what I call "my kids", the two dogs, Bella and Tuck.

Always looking for a life lesson, I started to teach my daughters as young women the importance of setting healthy boundaries. Teaching them that it's okay to make mistakes in order to learn and grow. That if we overreact to circumstances, we may miss the lesson, the gift.

Like many women my next steps were learning self-love, placing value on myself and the novelty of being alone after many, many years of being married. I started to embrace the peace and tranquility of a quiet home, waking up each day feeling happy, refreshed, and grateful to start my day…knowing that this is exactly the way my life is supposed to be at this moment.

MY STORY: The Turning Point

At 49 years old, I woke up one morning and looked at the stranger in the mirror. I had lost control of my body. With all the stress in my life and divorce looming, I had stopped paying attention.

That moment was a jolt and the beginning of my journey.

Our relationship with our body is the influencer that establishes the quality and perceptions of our life experiences. Too often I hear from women that they've been told, 'Menopause is part of aging. Just accept it.'

Menopause is part of aging, but you don't have to just accept feeling confused, insecure, and not like yourself. You can feel like an informed participant in your own health and wellbeing. You can be the architect of your own plan. And I'm here to help you do that coming from a place of experience and empathy, without judgment.

In 2012, when I made another conscious investment in my wellbeing, I lost over 30 pounds and my whole personality changed with renewed confidence and heightened self-esteem.

During menopause I recognized the challenges women faced both physically and emotionally to move past their worst menopause symptoms. Unfortunately, not all women have the same experience as they cannot find the answers, they so desire, and often pass harsh judgement on their body image as a measure of self-worth.

As a woman my journey through menopause created many life challenges. As a scientist I spent hours researching and even reached back to my peers to find the answers I was desperately seeking. Once I found the secret, and had a sense of being in control, my experience changed, and my purpose became clear. My vision was to share the answers with women who were struggling as I had. My goal was to reach as many women as possible including an online presence for an even broader reach.

I recognize the strong link between hormone imbalance, self-image, self-esteem, and relationships. I open my heart to women to share my story and expertise to inspire them to strive for happiness in their own lives.

It's all about making peace with our body and having the confidence to take control back. Or maybe gain it for the first time.

In my 1:1 coaching with women, I encourage them not to give up; there are answers. At 59 years old, I still do everything possible to stay healthy and embrace my body with respect.

Why have I shared this with you? And why does this drive what I'm doing now?

My passion is working closely with women to support their transition through peri-menopause and menopause by creating a community of accountability and support. I encourage women to embrace a positive relationship with their body which in turn will attract positive life experiences. I want others to benefit from what I've learned and experienced. I've been through it, so I can be your 'expert guide' and make this journey easier.

As you begin to read this book, please make it an interactive event plus a time for your own reflection of some of the turning points and mentors in your life. My goal is to educate you, help you to finally find your true answers and set you on the path to defining your happiness. Menopause is a journey. Embrace it knowing you can find your true self and acknowledge the need for self-care.

Let's get started. I hope each of you will find something in these pages that resonates with you, gives you hope and helps you to grow as a woman in this chapter of your life, and to become the person you crave, to "Restore Your Life."

Your 'Why?'

Why are you reading this? What are you facing? What do you feel are your roadblocks? What would you change in your life right now if you could? Answer these questions before you proceed. Be honest and true to yourself to accept your own perspective of your life as it is with the desire to make changes!

I've shared a bit about me, and some major events and turning points in my life. I want you to understand my motivation and see that I have been on a journey to get where I am today. It wasn't a straight line, even though the young me thought it would work out that way. There were twists along the way, some surprises, and a point where my life path ended on one track but began again on another.

Because of it, I feel I am a better, stronger, happier, healthier person. And because I am in such a good place, I feel the need to give back. I want to help women just like you as you navigate through pre/peri-menopause and menopause. I want you to feel more in control and to arrive in a better place than you ever imagined possible.

That's what drives me. That's my purpose. It's my WHY.

So, what's your why?

Why are you reading this?

I want you to find a few uninterrupted minutes for yourself, in a comfortable place, maybe with a cup of tea, maybe with your favourite music, with a pencil, and an open, loving mind.

What are you facing? What do you feel are roadblocks? What would you change in your life right now if you could?

_____

_____

_____

_____

Consider the following:

Am I feeling good / healthy right now?

_____

_____

_____

_____

What does 'good' feel like?

List the first three or four things you think of. Some suggestions to get you thinking: energetic, rested, happy, confident, desirable, in control.

_____

_____

_____

_____

What does healthy mean to you? Does it mean having an ailment under control, or the absence of medications? Does it mean being physically fit? Does it include a positive state of mind?

_____

_____

_____

_____

What are the roadblocks preventing you from feeling good and healthy? Is it a lack of time? Is it that other things are taking priority over your self-care?

_____

_____

_____

_____

Do you know what steps to take to make the changes you desire? Can you commit to self-care?

_____

_____

_____

_____

Please complete the **Menopause Symptom Checklist** before proceeding to the next chapter.

Review it each time you move forward to another chapter, so your symptoms are front of mind and your perception is clear. This will assist your learning specific to your needs and your ability to identify with the women you are about to meet.

The Menopause Symptom Checklist

You may wish to copy this checklist and revisit it every 3 to 6 months to see how your symptoms change over time.

Use this table to track the symptoms you are experiencing as:
0 (none), 1 (mild), 2 (moderate), 3 (severe)

				Date					
0	1	2	3	Hot flashes	0	1	2	3	Decreased muscle mass
0	1	2	3	Night sweats	0	1	2	3	Excess facial/body hair
0	1	2	3	Heart palpitations	0	1	2	3	Loss of scalp hair
0	1	2	3	Water retention	0	1	2	3	Increased acne
0	1	2	3	Cold body temp	0	1	2	3	Oily skin
0	1	2	3	Weight gain – waist	0	1	2	3	Muscle aches/ stiffness
0	1	2	3	Weight gain – hips	0	1	2	3	Bone loss
0	1	2	3	Sleep disturbances	0	1	2	3	Vaginal dryness
0	1	2	3	Low blood sugar	0	1	2	3	Incontinence
0	1	2	3	Allergies	0	1	2	3	Breast tenderness
0	1	2	3	Nausea	0	1	2	3	Fibrocystic breasts
0	1	2	3	Fatigue	0	1	2	3	Bleeding changes
0	1	2	3	Drowsiness	0	1	2	3	Uterine fibroids
0	1	2	3	Low sex drive	0	1	2	3	Breast swelling
0	1	2	3	Headaches	0	1	2	3	Feel 'pressed for time'
0	1	2	3	Feel 'tired but wired'	0	1	2	3	Unable to cope
0	1	2	3	Tearfulness	0	1	2	3	Poor exercise tolerance
0	1	2	3	Depression	0	1	2	3	Caffeine consumption
0	1	2	3	Mood swings	0	1	2	3	Morning sluggishness
0	1	2	3	Irritability	0	1	2	3	Memory lapses
0	1	2	3	Anxiety	0	1	2	3	Foggy thinking
0	1	2	3	Feel 'burned out'	0	1	2	3	

Note any major life changes or stressors that have happened around the time you are tracking your symptoms.

_____

_____

_____

_____

_____

_____

_____

_____

_____

_____

_____

_____

_____

_____

_____

_____

_____

_____

_____

_____

_____

_____

_____

_____

It's Not Your Fault.
No One Gives Us the Answers!

Through my own experience, I recognized that menopause can be very uncomfortable and frustrating; however, one of the many purposes of my book is to encourage women not to give up and let the symptoms rule your life. Don't let menopause define who you are. There are answers!

As a woman who has also struggled through menopause, I need to start this book by strongly affirming, "This is not your fault!!". Our biggest challenge in successfully transitioning through menopause is, NO ONE GIVES US THE ANSWERS and, if they do, it often leads us in the wrong direction.

Women will spend hours of frustration plus wasted dollars seeking information, reassurance, relief and, sometimes, quick fixes in desperation. They'll attempt solutions that just don't fit their circumstance or history, let alone their own personal body chemistry.

My story began while working diligently to accept a failed marriage and ultimate divorce, coupled with battling 'the change of life.' I am sure many of my readers have been down this road. Here I was, not looking, or feeling myself with my self-image hitting an ultimate low. I had to shift quickly to regain control of my changing body as well as my self-esteem.

I often look back all too clearly to that moment of realization when I woke up in the middle of the night with these intense night sweats. I was covered in sweat and my bed was soaked. I was mortified and I literally had no concept of what was happening to my body. Unfortunately, it started to happen night after night. My energy dropped dramatically. I was so exhausted. Every day became a struggle clouded with fatigue.

After one night, with barely a few hours' sleep, I got up in the morning and looked at myself in the mirror with fear and anxiety. Who was this stranger? I had lost all accountability for self-care. I wasn't paying attention. After all, my self-care didn't come first. Work, children, and a life full of responsibility to others always took precedence over me. I looked in the mirror with despair. I had lost the vibrancy in my eyes. I looked down at my tummy with disgust. I had unfortunately acquired the ultimate muffin-top well known to menopausal women across the world. My body shape had shifted dramatically along with my self-esteem. All of which contributed to low libido.

I looked at this woman in the mirror with awe. She was a complete and utter stranger to me. At 49, I was now in the early stages of menopause, and I had allowed the symptoms to take over my life.

As women we go through such intense changes in our body image as we transition through menopause. And it feels like it happens almost overnight. We look back at pictures and suddenly feel unrecognizable and often start to avoid social functions out of embarrassment.

I know how quickly it happens, or perhaps it is so gradual in the beginning it is unnoticeable. Perhaps we are just not paying attention. One day we wake up full of energy and ready to take on the challenges of the day, and then somehow, we have lost our energy, put on weight, our sex drive is gone, and we are stumbling around in a constant fog. Our personality has shifted. We don't even recognize this woman, struggling with embarrassing mood swings, over-reacting to the smallest of circumstances.

Even as a health care professional I didn't have all the answers in the beginning. I kind of knew what to expect, but still felt I was caught off guard. When the answers to my questions weren't easily accessible, I had to go back to the science I knew, including reaching out to my colleagues. In reality I had to become my own mentor.

As women we may seek out the advice and experiences of our friends and family who have experienced menopausal symptoms. Yet their experiences and solutions may not work for us because our body chemistry is different – even between mothers, daughters, and sisters. While the symptoms are similar the causes vary.

So naturally we go to our doctors for answers but then leave the office in frustration after being told it's part of aging. "Accept it."

Meet Colette, a 56-year-old woman, struggling with hot flashes, weight gain, low energy, and insomnia. Like many women all was well until she reached the five-year window and was suddenly pulled off her HRT (hormone replacement therapy) medication with no other solution offered as a substitute by her female family physician. After circling back multiple times to her physician, Colette threw up her hands in frustration. Thus began the long road of random research online and trial and error solutions. Like many women, Colette was lost in a crowd with mainstream, over-the-counter solutions such as Black Cohosh and unsustainable results... until we met.

I am not judging... I encourage people to do their own research. Yet where do we begin? As a pharmacist and scientist, I started to realize that doctors and traditional medicine absolutely didn't have the answers I was seeking. I had to advocate for myself and be open to a different type of medicine based on my knowledge and learning from past mentors such as Maria.

After many trials and tribulations, I discovered the secret - the secret to accurately testing and learning how our body chemistry changes during menopause and can be positively affected by tailored supplements in a very precise mix. The solution was not a generic 'herb of the month.' I had to discover through self-testing how the correct mix of supplements at therapeutic dosing could positively affect hormone levels and dramatically improve the way I felt on a day-to-day basis.

Through my own experience I recognized that menopause can be very uncomfortable and frustrating; however, one of the many purposes of my book is to encourage women not to give up and let the symptoms rule your life. Don't allow the symptoms and challenges of menopause to define you as a woman in the prime of your life. It doesn't have to be your story. It will absolutely be your challenge, but it can also be your win, and your success story as you break free.

Once I discovered the key to solving my own worst menopause symptoms, I realized I could not keep this information to myself. I had to share it with as many women as possible. This was and still is my life's mission and passion, to share my expertise and the key to ending women's struggles. I know so many women struggle, sadly even women in their early 60s.

For women it is recognizing that their chemistry has changed dramatically. Whatever is going on under the surface is different. And it's different for each woman. The cause of hot flashes, for example, varies greatly from woman to woman yet we all may assume it's due to non-existent estrogen. After reviewing hundreds of saliva tests, I would never assume estrogen is low as it is greatly affected by body fat and past medications such as long-term use of birth control pills.

About 75 percent of women experience hot flashes during menopause, making it the most common symptom experienced by menopausal women. Hot flashes can occur at any time, multiple times a day (or night). Many women will probably experience them to variable degrees over a period of years or longer.

Triggers for this sudden volcanic eruption of body heat from your chest, neck and face can include:

➢ consuming alcohol or caffeine

➢ eating spicy food

➢ feeling stressed or anxious

➢ being overweight

➢ overindulging in sugar

➢ being in a warm room

During this time of life, some women may also experience muscle and joint pain trying not to fall into the diagnosis of arthritis. Horrific mood swings can result in a change in personality making it difficult to determine whether these symptoms are caused by shifts in hormones, life circumstances, stress, or a combination of all three.

So, you visit your doctor with a list of complaints, seeking support, guidance, and relief. Instead, you leave with the advice that 'It's a part of aging, get used to it,' and a bag full of medications such as birth control pills, hormone therapy, anti-depressants, sleeping pills, blood pressure medication and more, leading at times to a long list of side-effects. A medicinal treatment plan that your body may not embrace as it works against our natural grain.

This can be a difficult moment for a woman who is already feeling at a loss. But it doesn't have to be this way. Menopause is a natural change. The goal is to embrace the changes with the understanding that there are always answers. There are answers that are as individual as you are.

Don't Give Up Hope.

Think of it like this: Your hormones are like a chemistry equation, constantly shifting with each decade until we reach menopause. Each decade brings us a new body, one we can accept and even embrace.

The chemistry equation is continuously evolving and sometimes it gets out of line. To take back control, we need to find the root cause of our menopausal symptoms and balance our hormones. Nothing changes unless we provide our body with a tailored foundation of support.

My message to women is to not give up. You can still have the body you want, it's just that the solutions must be customized to you. We don't have to just accept the worst changes as part of aging. Our goal should be to find inner harmony, an inner feeling of contentment with who we are and where life is taking us. Perhaps it's also a time to take a personal inventory.

Just remember - there are answers waiting for you. As you will see in the next chapter, the biggest step in preparation is supporting our Adrenal Glands.

Adrenal Fatigue: If Only We Knew!

Our adrenal glands are our best partners during menopause. Women in menopause will struggle with low energy and excessive fatigue. It is like a light switch that is suddenly turned off. Adrenal fatigue will set in firmly to different degrees depending on a woman's ability to manage stress, the inner balance of her hormones, and the energy of her immediate environment. Don't just hope for the best… be prepared!

As we age and transition through menopause, supporting the adrenal glands should become a priority. Unfortunately, no one tells us this and so the struggle begins as we desperately seek answers to our worst symptoms. If you search online for 'adrenal fatigue' you will see there is a medical diagnosis for 'adrenal insufficiency' which is confirmed by a blood test from the doctor. Adrenal Fatigue, however, is disputed by the medical community as it is not a disease state. As an Integrative Practitioner I teach clients that it is a real condition with real symptoms, not a medical diagnosis.

Our adrenal glands are a feisty organ system that sits on top of the kidneys and produces hormones that help regulate metabolism, immune system, blood pressure, hormone balance, response to stress and other essential functions. When everything is functioning well, you feel vibrant and energized, ready to take on all of life's challenges.

Symptoms of adrenal fatigue include being tired, having poor sleep, salt and sugar cravings, and needing stimulants like caffeine to get through the day. These symptoms are common to many people (including men) and do not point to anything specific. They also can occur as part of a normal, busy life, so it is easy to dismiss them.

Most women in menopause will struggle with low energy and excessive fatigue. It is like a light switch that is suddenly turned off and we must reach for that extra cup of coffee or afternoon carbohydrate to push through our tasks at hand. Adrenal fatigue will set in firmly to different degrees depending on a woman's ability to manage stress, the inner balance of her hormones, and the energy of her immediate environment, the intimate circle of family and friends around her.

Our adrenal glands are our best partner and support system to cope with stress from all aspects of life, emotionally and physically. They provide our body with resilience, energy, and endurance. As our ovaries slowly shut down, it is up to our adrenal glands to kick in and maintain women's hormone levels chronologically over time.

Let's Talk Science

Adrenaline increases your heart rate, elevates your blood pressure, and boosts energy supplies. Cortisol, the primary stress hormone, increases sugars (glucose) in the bloodstream, enhances your brain's use of glucose and increases the availability of substances that repair tissues – everything you would need in an emergency.

This complex natural alarm system also communicates with the brain regions that control mood, motivation, and fear.

But when stress is always part of your life and you constantly feel under attack, that readiness state of fight-or-flight always stays turned on.

Your adrenal glands continue to produce adrenaline and cortisol and you don't relax (such as in a troubled relationship with a child or partner, or when you're under the cloud of financial pressure). This long-term state of always being 'on' is what creates adrenal fatigue.

Imagine what that does to your body over time. Imagine what a heightened level of stress hormones does to your body's processes. You could be at increased risk of many health problems, including:

- ☐ Anxiety
- ☐ Depression
- ☐ Digestive problems
- ☐ Headaches
- ☐ Muscle tension and pain
- ☐ Heart disease, heart attack, high blood pressure and stroke
- ☐ Sleep problems
- ☐ Weight gain
- ☐ Memory and concentration impairment
- ☐ Breast cancer

Stress and our overwhelming responsibility to manage day-to-day life often leaves women unprepared for menopause, too depleted to take on its unpredictable adventures. Part of the reason is we set the bar too high for ourselves to perfectly manage a career and the home front. Before you know it, your worst fears are realized as other symptoms of menopause start to appear (weight gain, fatigue, mood swings, night sweats, hot flashes, lower libido, etc.) impacting your wellbeing, self-image and state of mind.

Even with self-care in place our tool kit may become depleted as what worked in the past suddenly no longer produces results. As our environment takes over, we may face unforeseeable stress that we cannot escape. Our life can change direction so quickly with unexpected divorce, changes at work beyond our control, or a sudden stream of health challenges.

To make it more challenging, no one really informs us or warns us to anticipate a dramatic shift in self-image, body shape, energy, and multiple other symptoms, so we are left to chance, guessing as to what is wrong with our rapidly changing bodies.

Even as a pharmacist and integrative practitioner, I had a lot of tools in place, yet was not fully prepared.

So, what's truly happening to our body? And why do we feel so out of control?

Two of the hormones managed by the adrenal glands that directly influence our menopausal journey are Cortisol and DHEA. Adrenal insufficiency refers to inadequate production of one or more of these hormones. Adrenal fatigue, however, can also be due to excessive production of Cortisol.

Cortisol is a steroid hormone, also made in the adrenal glands and then released into the blood. It helps control the body's use of fats, proteins, and carbohydrates; suppresses inflammation; regulates blood pressure; increases blood sugar; and can also decrease bone formation (more on cortisol in a later chapter).

DHEA is called the mother hormone. It is the building block for all other hormones. Sustaining healthy levels of DHEA prior to menopause will prepare our body to successfully maintain hormone levels over time and avoid unwanted symptoms. Or in the very least control the degree of our symptoms which can impact our ability to function professionally at work and comfortably in our intimate relationships at home.

When we are in equilibrium and our hormones are in balance, we feel well. When we are in an extended period of stress, our hormones are out of balance as our bodies try to cope with this heightened sense of needing to be prepared for something – fight or flight. It will vary for all women depending on their coping skills, environment, and mindset.

Always remember that no two women's journeys are identical as there are just too many variables such as: medical history, personal stress, environmental stress, level of nutrition, level of physical activity, sleep pattern, levels of inflammation, prescription intake, weight, use of alcohol and tobacco, and more.

As challenging as it may be, I always encourage women to start working on their self-care and putting themselves first. It starts by finding time to be quiet and tranquil to assess your stress levels and work towards making some adjustments in your routines. It would be a simple yet particularly crucial step towards supporting your adrenal glands.

Developing a relationship with our authentic selves is a great time investment.

Why is Supporting the Adrenal Glands a Top Priority?

Adrenal fatigue is a universal problem that appears in various bodily conditions—especially seen in women complaining of high fatigue. It is usually caused by moderate and severe forms of stress and is commonly seen in women during menopause struggling with low or high cortisol levels.

Meet Heather, an executive with a career full of extreme responsibility and long hours. At 58 years old, her day often started at 7:00 a.m. due to their US partners. She was very active on the home front, entertaining, plus enjoying travel with her husband. She knew how to balance it all until she hit menopause and started to struggle with lack of sleep, night sweats, extreme daytime fatigue, poor food choices, and often using food and drink as stimulants.

Her signs and symptoms of adrenal fatigue varied from difficulty getting up in the morning, to memory loss, body aches and decreased productivity. Her fatigue was so high she often had to pull over to the side of the road for a power nap on her way to work.

After many visits to the doctor, she was offered sleeping pills and told that Adrenal Fatigue was a lay term, not a diagnosis. While her doctor was correct, she offered Heather little hope for her collection of non-specific symptoms. As those symptoms became overwhelming, Heather's body was unable to manage her stress and keep up with the level of demands in her life.

By the time Heather and I met she was consumed with fatigue and frustration, as are many women her age. As a no-nonsense business-person who expected results, she began with the Saliva Hormone Test to get a clear picture of her situation. Within weeks she was on the road to recovery as her symptoms quickly started to resolve after months of suffering. Her tailored solutions consisted of natural supplements specifically targeted and dosed to marry to her test results.

As Heather explained, it's easy to dismiss these feelings/experiences, attribute them to other causes, hope they'll just resolve themselves, or prioritize other things (and people) ahead of them. It's what women often do. However, if you are experiencing menopause with multiple unmanageable symptoms there may be a link to your adrenal gland. Once we understand the link and, more importantly, how to provide our body with support, we can make appropriate choices, and transition more easily along the menopause journey. As you will learn in the next chapter the beginning starts with a simple saliva hormone test to create a road map to follow along our menopause journey.

Adrenal Fatigue Checklist

Is this you…?

- ☐ Excessive morning sluggishness and fatigue
- ☐ High level of irritability and mood swings
- ☐ "Wired but tired"
- ☐ Unwanted and sudden weight gain
- ☐ Cravings for stimulants such as salt, sugar, caffeine
- ☐ General anxiety and heart palpitations
- ☐ Digestive problems
- ☐ Excess bloating
- ☐ Low levels of motivation
- ☐ Muscle wasting

The Secret Blueprint
for Menopause

There is a way to move past our worst menopausal symptoms and find tranquility and peace on the other side. Our chemistry is unique, and it reveals a personal blueprint that provides the road map for our menopause journey. Once I discovered the key, I was committed to sharing the 'secret' with as many women as possible.

As a woman of 59 years old and a women's health expert, I recognize that menopause is a natural journey all women will go through; however, not all women will experience it the same way. Life is not a cookie cutter. There are common symptoms, but not every woman will suffer from each one, or to the same degree. There is however a way to move past our worst menopausal symptoms and find tranquility on the other side.

As our chemistry is unique, a personal blueprint, not all women should be offered the same treatment plan. Unfortunately, that is not the way traditional medicine works. But in my experience – and probably yours – that's exactly the way it happens. Women often get no answers, the wrong answers, or the same cookie cutter treatments.

Let me share Lorraine's story. Lorraine was a 55-year-old woman struggling through menopause with symptoms of anxiety, hair loss, vaginal dryness, and low libido. Over the last four years she had visited her GP twice, a gynecologist, and two naturopaths, almost begging for assistance. According to all these doctors there were no answers for her! She was becoming very frustrated and disheartened at 'off the shelf' approaches for a very individual experience. In fact, she feared that something was very wrong. To her, menopause had become an illness.

I listened intently as Lorraine shared how she was feeling – physically and emotionally – delighted to finally have her concerns heard. Are these normal symptoms, she asked? It certainly wasn't close to what her mother had described. Was she in disease state? Some friends were struggling with the idea that this was the end of their childbearing years and therefore a loss of womanhood. Lorraine never felt that way. She looked forward to not having to worry about periods and birth control. But hair loss and low libido…? Was it going to get worse…? What should she expect next…? Were her feelings normal? No one was able to give her satisfactory answers or tailored solutions. Where would it end, she wondered?

Let me be clear: It's important for women to recognize it's not their fault. Even as a scientist, I struggled to get good solid information to understand my own experience through menopause and find the best solutions. Our healthcare system is just not set up to support this stage of a woman's life, so we just suffer through it, usually alone, and often give up.

Many women come up against roadblocks when seeking information and resources during menopause. Even for myself as a health care practitioner it took a lot of research to find my answers. I had to go back to the science I knew so well, including reaching out to my colleagues. My answers also came from some of the mentors in my life.

Once I found the key, the Saliva Hormone Test kit, and experienced the benefits firsthand, I had to share the secret with as many women as I could reach. My mission in life became to educate and support women as an expert guiding their transition through menopause, to minimize those feelings of frustration and disappointment as much as possible, with the ultimate goal of successfully resolving their worst menopausal symptoms, but also with the understanding that every day may not be perfect.

Lorraine talked and I just listened. When she was ready, we talked about hormones. Most of us learned about hormones when we went through puberty and were reminded of their power every month when we were premenstrual. Perimenopause and menopause are about hormones, too. Understanding them and their influence on our bodies and emotions can help provide clarity during this stage of life. Understanding is our way of taking control back and is a powerful first step.

I explained to Lorraine that it all starts with a saliva hormone test, an objective measure of your own unique body chemistry. By taking a simple test, you can learn exactly where your hormone levels are now, a picture of a moment in time and what is impacting the dramatic changes you are experiencing through menopause.

While there are blood tests that can measure hormones, I prefer the non-invasive and more accurate saliva test. The results provide a clear picture over time of what's been changing in your body below the surface. With the knowledge of that 'blueprint', you can be provided with tailored solutions - unique to you - to regulate your hormone levels. Within a short period of time, you will start to enjoy a greater sense of wellbeing and a healthier lifestyle with a very targeted dose-specific regimen of natural supplements based on your test results.

Your best choice is to embrace a multi-targeted program to support all five hormones, if necessary, and most importantly, the adrenal gland!

Here are the five key benefits to the innovative Saliva Hormone Test:

1. **Accuracy:** Saliva versus blood testing is much more accurate because it provides a clear picture of what's occurred over time at the cellular level, not just what's moving in and out of our bloodstream at the moment the lab draws blood.

2. **Convenience:** The Saliva Hormone Test is completed within five minutes in the comfort of your own home - no lab, no line-ups, no needles.

3. **Ease of Use:** The Saliva Hormone test is easy to use. You do it first thing in the morning prior to your morning coffee. Simply fill the vial with a small sample of saliva, complete the requisition

form (three minutes), freeze the sample, and call the courier. You'll get your results usually within 10 business days.

4. **Patient Specific**: The test provides you with a very specific blueprint that is unique to you! It will help you understand the exact reasons why you are experiencing so many symptoms… not the least of which is weight gain and the inability to release weight through methods that may have worked for you in the past.

5. **Thoroughness**: The Saliva Hormone Test includes the five key hormones that are specific to women experiencing menopause - Estradiol, Progesterone, Testosterone, DHEA and morning Cortisol.

These five hormones control hot flashes, brain fog, vaginal dryness, insomnia, muscle fatigue, stress, weight gain, anxiety, mood swings, the adrenal gland function, and much more.

This is all the information required to create a precise – and personalized – plan of action, all found in one simple test!

In the back of the book, "Developing Your Integrative Plan", I will discuss the case studies of seven amazing women, "The Girls." You will learn a little science in what their tests reveal and how this template guided their customized integrative plan. Remember, we are all individuals and it's important that our integrative plans are always created with this in mind. While their programs may look similar, dosages, uniqueness of the individual, and the targeted direction of the programs will vary.

Back to Lorraine….

Once Lorraine received her personal report on her hormone levels, identifying what was within normal ranges and what was 'out of whack' we walked through the report together. I explained to her how hormones were contributing to her symptoms and drew up a customized tailored regimen of natural supplements to address each one of her concerns.

Before I had her saliva test results, I had listened to Lorraine and reassured her that what she was experiencing was not unusual. In fact, her symptoms were mainstream to most women in menopause. However, it wasn't until I had the lab results that I developed Lorraine's Plan.

Without the precise information pointing her program in the right direction, anything I offered would have been the same old 'off the shelf' advice she had already received over the last four years - inaccurate, over the counter, under-dosed and poorly targeted programs.

Menopause Symptom Tracker

Tracking your symptoms and challenges over the next few weeks is crucial to you getting clarity, personalized advice, and guidance on how to best get past your worst menopause symptoms. Please complete these easy questions daily.

You may wish to copy this page for repeat use.

	S	M	T	W	T	F	S
Was it difficult to fall asleep last night?							
Did you experience a hormonal wake-up between 2am and 4am?							
Did you wake up last night?							
Did you experience night sweats?							
Do you feel energized and alert this morning?							
Did you have any hot flashes during the day?							
Any brain fog or lack of clarity?							
How was your mood today?							
Any anxiety, irritability or big mood swings?							
Rank your joint pain from 1 – 10 (10 being worst)							
Did you have low energy in the afternoon that caused you to reach for sugar or caffeine?							

Worksheet:
5 WAYS TO BEAT MENOPAUSE FATIGUE

Fatigue during menopause can dramatically affect your quality of life. Here are some tips and tools to work towards restoring your energy levels.

1. Exercise

Regular exercise is a great tool to combat fatigue and it also lowers Cortisol levels. Moderate to high intensity exercise is directly linked to higher energy levels. Remember, exercise can also trim fat, reduce hot flashes, and improve joint pain. Schedule exercise 3 to 5 times a week for 30 minutes. (Adding a 10-minute walk is a bonus) Pick an activity you enjoy and turn exercise into a habit!

My commitment:

_____

_____

_____

_____

_____

_____

_____

2. Sleep Routine

A good sleep routine can leave us feeling restored and energized. Go to bed and wake up at the same time every day, including weekends. Avoid alcohol and caffeine after dinner. Consider a warm shower, and avoid screen time (phone, tablet, computer, TV) for an hour prior to bed.

My commitment:

_____

_____

_____

_____

3. Meditate

It is surprising what a powerful tool meditation can be to improve sleep. Meditation can not only enhance sleep it also can lower stress levels. Choose a meditation that speaks to you for 5 minutes minimum prior to bed and sit quietly to clear your mind. Our best success is to have structure and routine to have the maximum benefit with meditation.

My commitment:

_____

_____

_____

_____

4. Turn down the thermostat

Keeping your room cool at night accommodates your body's natural temperature fluctuations. Ideal temperature for a good sleep is 65F (18C). In addition, avoid sugar and alcohol before bed as they will spike body temperature during the night. It can also cause unwanted weight gain and belly fat due to spiking of blood sugar during the night.

My commitment:

_____

_____

_____

_____

5. Downsize your meals

Eating a smaller meal in the evening will cause less bloating and possible discomfort during the night. Eating smaller portions of a healthy choice of vegetables and protein and low carbohydrates will also balance blood sugar overnight. Mixed kale with chicken, for example, is an easy choice with very minimal preparation.

My commitment:

_____

_____

_____

_____

The Integrative Practitioner:
MY STORY

As I began to blend my knowledge as a pharmacist with the practice of Integrative Medicine, I suddenly realized it was a very logical approach – a holistic medical approach that considers the lifestyle habits of the client and treats them as a whole person.

Meeting the right mentors along the way helped me to transition to a different type of medicine, offering my clients the best of both worlds. This is my story!

The Integrative Practitioner

As I started to learn more about the history and practice of Integrative Medicine, and how it places the individual at the centre of care, rather than the symptom or disease, I suddenly realized it was a very logical approach. It's a holistic medical approach that considers the lifestyle habits of a client and treats them as a whole person, not an isolated issue or complaint.

At that time, I met my second mentor, an Herbalist extremely intelligent in her practice with the background of a scientist, like myself. I started to learn more about our mind-body connection and how our emotional health is connected to our physical health. In addition, I realized all the pieces to the health and well-being puzzle include proper nutrition, moderate exercise, stress management, releasing old habits that no longer serve us, maintaining a positive mindset, morning structure and much more. As I learned, "Strong women eat well and embrace all aspects of their wellness."

By then, I had invested years in post secondary studies and had 10 years' experience as a professional pharmacist. However, life and the choices we make to support our health are not black and white. This was the beginning of my transition to following a new pathway of learning and embracing Integrative Medicine. I started to build a client base practicing my new skills. I even entertained the idea of cancelling my pharmacist licence, but I recognized the credibility of marrying the two worlds of pharmaceuticals and natural medicine. It certainly added to my clients' attraction, trust, and faith in working directly with me, as I was often told.

The more I learned about Integrative Medicine the more excited I became at the possibilities. I recognized there was another way to logically support our health and it made so much sense.

I started to think more and more about moving away from the pharmaceutical industry. As my new skills grew and I started to unleash my expertise, I recognized I could teach clients to support their health with a much more efficient and logical approach.

As I crossed the threshold to yet another type of medicine, of course women's health was always my focus and passion. Eventually I opened Avita Integrative Health Clinic and Compounding Lab in September 2009 to put into practice my new knowledge and skills in Bio-Identical Compounding alongside the Saliva Hormone Test.

Natural vs. Bio-Identical Hormones

The first step to frame your journey is the saliva hormone test, and the second step is to determine the best treatment options based on your unique chemistry. Marrying the saliva test to your health profile and medical history provides a guided road map....and so the journey begins.

From my perspective as an expert, the client has three options:

1. bio-identical hormones
2. natural supplements (my preference), or
3. a combination of both.

It all depends on the saliva test results, as you will see in further chapters!

Unfortunately, not having the answers they were seeking at their fingertips and desperate for relief, women may travel the road of pharmaceuticals, seeking a better quality of life. Bio-identical hormone creams became popular due to the lessening of side effects compared to traditional pharmaceuticals which women were fearful of. In 2008, bio-identical hormones became a very hot topic, even being promoted by celebrities.

As a pharmacist I always believed in the value of maintaining my knowledge as a source of credibility to my clients. In 2007, I was still working very part-time at a large Canadian chain pharmacy when I met another life-altering mentor, Carol, a pharmacy technician and, more importantly, teacher of the pharmacy technician program at a local college. As I listened to Carol passionately discuss the limitless possibilities with compounding my interest was piqued. Soon after, I spent a week training in Texas at the PCCA facility.

Feeling proud of my accomplishment and banking on my husband's support, instead my 25-year marriage was soon coming to an end. I remember feeling so disappointed and sad. Despite my growing knowledge and ability to provide care, in my eyes my personal life was a failure. My marriage was in a very dark place. And I walked that journey alone, mortified, and fearful of the outcome for my four children. I hid my secret, kept my game face on and continued to push forward in my career.

Prior to opening my own clinic and compounding lab I had been working alongside a family doctor treating his clients with Integrative Medicine and very customized, tailored solutions following saliva hormone testing. Clients were provided with three choices depending on the road map of their Saliva Hormone Test. For some women bio-identical hormones were never an option if their hormone levels were high, which often shocked them. This is another myth of menopause as most women will assume all their hormones become depleted during menopause. (Without proper testing women may start to incorporate Phytoestrogens into their diet and may actually put themselves in harm's way, especially if they are estrogen dominant).

Back to compounding... my frustration at that time was outsourcing the bio-identical hormones to other pharmacies with little to no control on quality assurance. As I was about to learn, compounding was quite an art as well as a science.

Combining my medicinal knowledge along with the integrative practitioner was powerful. I started to embrace women's journeys through menopause as my own, having walked in their shoes. It culminated in 2009, when I proudly opened Avita Integrative Health, an integrative clinic with a beautiful compounding lab. Sharing my knowledge and expertise as a woman and a pharmacist, my practice quickly gained heightened awareness and momentum.

I started to teach my clients the benefits of the bio-identical hormones working with custom-made hormone creams tailored according to their chemistry.

The term bio-identical means hormones identical in structure to those your body produces. In theory they fit like a lock and key into our receptors with little to no side effects as your body recognizes them as their own. The hormones in bioidentical medications are different from those in traditional hormone therapies, much safer, with less tendency to produce side effects. However, they are classified as drugs.

The term 'natural' means the powdered ingredients are sourced from plant or animal; they're not synthesized in a lab from animal by-products or other chemicals. For example, desiccated thyroid powder for hypothyroidism is from a bovine source and Natural Progesterone is sourced from wild yam. Over time drug companies also started to manufacture bio-identical hormones in fixed dosages, not the best choice for everyone. Conversely, compounded bio-identical hormones are custom made by a pharmacist, directed by the template of the Saliva Hormone Test. This process is known as compounding.

Compounding typically involves ingredients being combined and tailored to meet the specific needs and chemistry of an individual, in my opinion a much more proficient and beneficial process for the client. The possibilities for compounding are limitless and very tailored to the client's needs.

The hormones in bio-identical hormone replacement therapy (BHRT) are different from those used in traditional hormone replacement therapy (HRT) in that they're identical chemically to those our bodies produce naturally and are made from compounds found in plants, such as soyabeans or wild yam. The hormones used in traditional HRT are made from the urine of pregnant horses and other synthetic hormones thus creating the side effects and dangers as pointed out by the Women's Health Study (WHIS).

Hormones are very powerful and affect every tissue in our body, either directly or indirectly. It goes way beyond simply supplementing with estrogen, specifically Premarin, and progesterone, such as Provera, which forces non-human hormones into our body putting us in distress. While 50 percent of estrogen in Premarin is bio-identical, there are hundreds of non-human hormones and by-products. As I always explain to clients, it's not so much the drug that produces the side effects, it's the metabolites that can persist and build up in our body for years depending on our ability to eliminate them. For example, if a client suffers from constipation this can make the buildup of toxins even greater.

The bottom line is that a body in distress signals that side effects have kicked in due to the accumulation of a drug. One way to overcome this is by detoxifying with herbs, specifically targeting the organs of elimination: kidney/bladder, liver, and colon.

The findings of the WHIS highlighted that the long-term side effects of prescribing both Premarin and Provera together was increased risks of heart disease, breast cancer, stroke, blood clots and dementia. Surprisingly, using Premarin alone had less significant side effects (not that this protocol is ideal to alleviating symptoms of menopause) than the combination with Provera. Although there is substantial increased risk of stroke with Premarin, my suggestion is to avoid both at all costs. For a period of time Premarin had a black box warning from Health Canada yet was still available in pharmacies. Now it is dispensed as if the WHIS never occurred. A very unsettling situation for women.

At the end of the WHIS study we learned the importance of delivering the correct hormones, in the correct dosages, with the best delivery system. In the case of BHRT, creams delivered through the skin is best way to avoid the passage of medication through the liver. It is always best to start at lower dosages and monitor the client's success than to start high. Starting high means there is a risk of the drug accumulating in the skin; plus, everyone's skin absorbs at a different rate of bioavailability.

(Bioavailability is the fraction of administered drug that reaches our blood stream and systemic circulation).

Let's Talk About Progesterone

Over time the critical difference between synthetic Progestins and natural Progesterone became forgotten by the medical community, putting women at extremely high risk. Progestins do not have the same effect as Progesterone on other body tissues, only the endometrium (the inner lining of the uterus). Progestins, for example, are harmful during pregnancy. Unfortunately, physicians started to use them interchangeably.

This carelessness allowed the medical community to promote and highlight Progestins in women's treatment plans to have similar benefits to BHRT. Very far from the truth and creating more harm as this protocol evolved. Partnering it with Premarin was the biggest error as pointed out by the WHIS.

In the end it made much more sense to stick with either true BHRT, therapeutic herbal supplements, or a combination of both.

Bear in mind our best course of treatment is mapped out by the individual blueprint of the saliva hormone test as discussed in previous chapters, as it gives us an exact picture of each woman's chemistry.

BHRT is typically used as women age and hormone levels shift, particularly for women who are in perimenopause or menopause. It's used to increase the levels of the hormones that have dropped and improve moderate to severe menopause symptoms including:

- ☐ hot flashes
- ☐ mood swings or irritability
- ☐ brain fog
- ☐ weight gain
- ☐ low libido
- ☐ night sweats
- ☐ memory loss
- ☐ joint pain
- ☐ insomnia
- ☐ vaginal dryness and/or painful intercourse

However, as outlined earlier, sometimes hormone levels may be high making BHRT a non-option in a treatment protocol.

In addition to helping with menopausal symptoms, there is some evidence that BHRT may also reduce your risk of disease states such as diabetes, hypertension, and high cholesterol. From an aesthetic perspective there is also some proof that it can help improve thinning of the skin, hydration, elasticity, and even reduce wrinkles. Yet, I have also worked with many women surprised to see all these improvements with the correct therapeutic dosages of herbs (for example improvements in the thinning of the vaginal walls without a messy cream!).

So, What Does a Bio-Identical Plan Look Like?

While there are many benefits to BHRT and HRT, it may not be the right choice for everyone, for personal or medical reasons. For example, some medical conditions such as a history of breast cancer may prevent you from safely being able to use it, or you may choose not to use that form of treatment for personal reasons or beliefs. Often fear of side effects is at the forefront.

Many women cannot take BHRT or any form of hormone replacement. For other women BHRT or HRT has proven to be highly effective in improving their general well-being and quality of life. It can be a very euphoric effect as their body embraces the support, especially if certain hormones are depleted (as you will see when you meet Sandra in a later chapter). However, the risks don't change. The potential for side effects will vary among women depending on their health history.

I never judge a woman's choice as it is their journey and at times the suffering is overwhelming. Perhaps they simply crave a normalcy that allows their mind to disregard the risk of side effects. Perhaps they desperately crave to get their body back along with their self-esteem.

As a pharmacist I observed the benefits of bio-identical hormones firsthand as I saw it in many clients I treated. The advantage of the bio-identical hormones is their exact match in structure to our own natural hormones, therefore, far fewer side effects as the body recognizes them as their own and fit like a lock and key into our receptors.

Being an integrative practitioner, however, and a big believer in the power of natural supplements, I had never entertained the treatment for myself. Plus, from a natural perspective, I always encouraged lifestyle changes along with prescribed supplements as a first line treatment to help reduce the intensity of women's menopausal symptoms including:

- ☐ moderate exercise
- ☐ weight release
- ☐ avoidance of foods that aggravate symptoms such as sugar, caffeine and alcohol
- ☐ embracing a sustainable, reasonable lifestyle
- ☐ reducing carbohydrates
- ☐ implementing a structured morning routine of self-care
- ☐ journaling
- ☐ meditation
- ☐ acupuncture or other modalities to reduce stress levels

While these measures would not eliminate all symptoms it certainly provided the client with a well-rounded treatment and daily structure. Even herbs are best taken with the above lifestyle modifications to provide more than one pillar of support.

The Compounding Pharmacist

Developing my skill as a compounder required ongoing training to enhance my knowledge base. It also meant many trips to the US for specialized training to continue to grow and develop my skill. As a practitioner, having the Saliva Hormone Kit in my tool bag was an advantage for both myself and my clients. Seeing the positive change in hormone levels during treatment, along with their diminishing symptoms, certainly gave the client confidence that we were on the right pathway.

In time, I did start to recognize that more women were leaning towards utilizing the herbs/natural supplements in therapeutic dosages matching the map of their saliva hormone test. I was always proud and fortunate not to be on any medication, choosing the natural supplements above all else, understanding however that the supplements were not a cookie cutter and had to be dosed appropriately.

I believe the shift to natural medicine began once women recognized it as a very individualized, client-centred model of promoting optimal health and wellness, combining a whole person approach with evidence-based strategies to reduce disease risk by turning around lifestyle behaviours.

It doesn't just treat the disease, if applicable, but actually works to prevent disease in the first place. The mind, body and soul of the client were all taken into consideration to promote healing and wellbeing.

Integrative Medicine actively places the client in a much more powerful position than in conventional medicine as they can make decisions on their own based on the options provided, becoming the director of their health. It connects all the dots and puts all choices available on the table, such as proper nutrition, lifestyle modification, exercise, stress management, regular structured habits and much more, embracing all the immediate health concerns and symptoms collectively.

I became very motivated and encouraged as I was able to put the individual client at the centre of care, addressing all areas of their health. Not the isolated, disconnected, one problem at a time approach their physician always used.

As a pharmacist and integrative practitioner, I became very successful at safely integrating medication with herbs, if required. I was very proud of the fact that I was offsetting the side effects of the medication and was often able to work with the client and their physician to decrease dosages or eliminate medication altogether from the client's roster.

While I was experiencing joy and growth as I diligently built a practice and raised my children, I wasn't paying close attention to all aspects of my life. In 2011, there was a simultaneous explosion in my life and my marriage dissolved. I knew there was an important lesson; however, at first, I was too blinded by hurt and disappointment to perceive the good. Again, I felt very alone and scared for myself and my children, worried I would lose all my financial stability.

Feeling stuck it took time for me to plan my next steps while trying desperately to find a way out. In addition, at that time I was very unhappy with my body image, another aspect I had not been paying attention to.

I jumped into the Avita Weight Loss System (I became my own client!) with no expectations or goals except to lose the unwanted weight. Everything lined up for me. I lost over 30 lbs., regained my self-esteem and found the courage I needed to embrace the new chapter in my life. I happily divorced in 2012 finding the strength to move forward.

I re-entered the world refreshed, happy to dive deep into my business as an Integrative Practitioner and continue to support women's health. The bio-identical hormones I dispensed were very successful, yet I felt unaligned due to my passion for integrative medicine. Women sought out my services embracing the opportunity to work with not only a health care professional and women's health expert, but a woman who had experienced menopause firsthand. The Saliva Hormone Test was a strong tool to provide the blueprint to customize solutions. There was a science behind the compounding of the creams, multi-targeted and dosed according to the saliva test results.

My discomfort was the necessity over time to increase dosages to attain the same results and resolution of unwanted menopausal symptoms. The necessity to increase hormone dosages was driven by the client's tolerance to the drug, as is common with many medications. With the herbs, however, dosages slowly decreased over time once the client reached their optimum peak of health. The recommendation was a 3-month window of herbs at therapeutic dosages where clients would experience many far-reaching benefits in addition to balancing their hormone system.

Fast forward to 2019 and the compounding lab at Avita Integrative Health was 10 years old. My lease was up for renewal and the opportunity to make a change in my business presented itself. I decided it was time to narrow down my offering and re-align my vision. I followed my passion which was working specifically with women in menopause for weight release and hormone balancing. However, I decided to work only with natural supplements to multi-target their hormone system. The universe was shifting at that time, and I found fewer women were seeking bio-identical hormones, preferring the natural support of high-grade herbal supplements.

In August 2019, the compounding lab sold, and I moved my pharmacist licence to the retired list after more than 30 years. I was able to focus on my expertise in women's health through the modality of integrative medicine with 25-plus years' experience both personally and professionally. Avita Integrative Health had already expanded to four locations in the Greater Toronto Area specializing in saliva hormone testing and customized solutions for menopause, often with the added service of weight loss. Life was very busy!

My business goal by the end of 2020 was to be online with the intent that I could travel and run my business from anywhere in the world. However, I was procrastinating due to my discomfort with technology and social media. When the pandemic hit in March 2020 my hand was forced. I chose to close all four clinics and embraced the opportunity to pivot online and fulfil my dream. I began to accept the online world, sharing my expertise and meeting an amazing group of women who otherwise never would have entered my circle. Many had been struggling for years to find the answers they were desperately seeking to overcome their worst menopausal symptoms. I became a teacher and mentor openly discussing their options. If there was a desire to use the bio-identical hormones I was not here to judge but to guide them with my knowledge and expertise. I could still utilize my training as a compounder without the stress and responsibility of dispensing.

Without diminishing the fact that COVID-19 has had devastating effects on many people, for me the Covid situation was a motivator that prompted me to pivot online, reaching a much broader audience of women, sharing my expertise with authenticity and compassion, building nurturing relationships with women to support and guide their menopause journey! From my perspective and experience this also meant 1:1 coaching for women to create structure and self-care in their lives by putting #1 first.

Unfortunately, I wasn't practising what I was preaching, putting myself last. As you will see in upcoming chapters, controlling and managing our stress is a crucial piece of self-care as, without it, it can lower our defences and impair our ability to manage disease.

Is Your Thyroid Off Balance?

You present the following symptoms: rapid weight gain, fatigue, consti-pation, hoarseness, increased sensitivity to cold. Your thyroid test comes back negative, yet the symptoms persist. Is it menopause or hypothyroidism? Perhaps it's both… let me explain the science.

After struggling for months, you seek out the advice of your family doctor, worried that maybe your thyroid is out of balance. You present the following symptoms:

- ☐ rapid weight gain
- ☐ fatigue
- ☐ constipation
- ☐ hoarseness
- ☐ increased sensitivity to cold

Your doctor rolls his eyes and says this is simple. You're aging! And probably eating all the wrong foods. Your eyes well up with tears and you beg for a thyroid panel. Begrudgingly, he agrees to test TSH alone. Test results come back positive for hypothyroidism, and he puts you on Synthroid 'for life.' Is this your story? I have heard it many, many times!

Months go by and you see no improvements. Fearful of your doctor's response you instead seek information and advice wherever you can find it, thinking that perhaps thyroid imbalance goes hand-in-hand with menopause, or that it all starts with thyroid imbalance leading to menopause.

The confusion begins. Is it early menopause or is your thyroid out of balance?

I believe our 50s is a time to be cherished. Our career is at its peak, kids are leaving the nest, and finally we can pay attention to our own self-care. Then suddenly the symptoms start to kick in. Your body is gaining seemingly uncontrollable weight, your mind is clouded and foggy. Your doctor tells you your cholesterol is high even though your nutrition is on the mark, and you exercise regularly. Your mood swings are erratic, often making you feel out of control - almost like a split personality. You're exhausted by mid-afternoon, reaching for more caffeine to power through yet at night you struggle with insomnia. Your libido is in the dumpster even though you are still deeply in love with your partner. Your hair is falling out in chunks and your thermostat fluctuates from hot to cold.

Sadly, most women will struggle with fluctuating hormones for four to eight years or longer before hitting post-menopause. And still the struggle continues if we are not providing our body with a foundation of support.

Desperate for relief you grasp for hope, trying treatment after treatment. You may start with the herb of the month mentality and purchase black cohosh. When that has limited or no results you may jump onto the trendy treatment of bio-identical hormones. Your last resort is your physician who may prescribe HRT (hormone replacement therapy) leaving you in a fog of fear for the side effects and increased risk of breast cancer.

While some of these treatments may provide results (or simply mask your symptoms in the short term), the issue is the thyroid and the adrenal gland need to be targeted together. Remember, all the cards need to be put on the table and simultaneously treated for top results and utmost resolution of unwanted symptoms to live the life you so desire. So, let's discuss the thyroid.

The thyroid is the butterfly-shaped organ in your throat. It is the master of our metabolism and energy affecting almost every organ in your body. Like a computer it is the control panel that regulates the body's metabolism and all the chemical reactions in your body. It also secretes several hormones:

> Thyroxine (T4)

> Triiodothyronine (T3)

> Calcitonin

The multi-faceted function of the thyroid is directly linked to a woman's reproductive system and menstrual cycle. As it relates to menopause, an imbalance in thyroid hormone levels may cause the early onset of menopause and adrenal fatigue (before age 40 or in the early 40s). This is often missed or under-diagnosed by physicians.

Early signs of thyroid problems include: (see also a more comprehensive low and high thyroid checklist in the back of the book)

☐ gastrointestinal problems

☐ mood changes

☐ weight changes

☐ skin problems

☐ sensitivity to temperature changes

☐ vision changes (occurs more often with hyperthyroidism)

☐ hair thinning or hair loss (hyperthyroidism)

☐ memory problems (both hyperthyroidism and hypothyroidism)

Hyperthyroidism means your thyroid gland is too active. The thyroid is making more thyroid hormones than it needs to, making your metabolism work at a faster rate.

Hyperthyroidism may occur for several reasons including Grave's disease, toxic nodular goiter, and thyroiditis, but can also be caused by taking too much thyroid hormone medicine to treat an underactive thyroid, having too much iodine in your diet, or having a growth in the pituitary gland that makes your thyroid overactive.

Symptoms may include:

- ☐ nervousness
- ☐ irritability
- ☐ sensitivity to heat
- ☐ extra sweating (perspiration), and
- ☐ fine, brittle hair.

Left untreated, hyperthyroidism can cause serious heart problems and brittle bones.

Hypothyroidism is the most common type of thyroid disorder. It means your thyroid gland is not active enough. When your thyroid doesn't make enough hormones, parts of your body slow down, especially your metabolism.

It is the most common thyroid condition I have seen in my practice. The saliva hormone test is important as many hormones are affected by our thyroid and vice versa. For example, high estradiol can block thyroid function. In addition, balanced Cortisol is required for proper conversion of T4 to T3 which can affect the success of Synthroid.

Some symptoms of underactive thyroid may be mistaken for early menopause, thus being proactive with proper testing is key, including both a thyroid panel and a saliva hormone test. Signs may include lack of menstruation, hot flashes, insomnia, and mood swings. Treating hypothyroidism can sometimes ease symptoms of early menopause or prevent early menopause from happening.

The most common cause of hypothyroidism is an autoimmune disorder (Hashimoto's disease), meaning your immune system starts to attack itself by making antibodies against the thyroid gland. Another cause may be treatment for an overactive thyroid with radioactive iodine therapy or thyroid removal.

The medical intervention with Hashimoto's disease can vary. I have treated clients supported with Synthroid and some without. As an Integrative Practitioner my goal, of course, is always to treat the whole body, supporting thyroid, liver, adrenal gland, and the sex hormones (estradiol and progesterone), putting the body into a foundational state of detoxification.

Targeting the thyroid alone will never be enough to produce the desired results or to address the health concerns as presented. The degree of symptoms varies and are different for each person. They may be hard to notice at first, starting slow and steady, and may often be mistaken for symptoms of depression.

Many, many women face these symptoms. Does this sound familiar?

- ☐ Tiredness (fatigue)
- ☐ Sensitivity to cold
- ☐ Hoarse voice
- ☐ Slow speech
- ☐ Droopy eyelids
- ☐ Puffy face
- ☐ Weight gain
- ☐ Constipation
- ☐ Sparse, coarse, and dry hair
- ☐ Dry skin and brittle nails
- ☐ Hand tingling or pain
- ☐ Slow pulse
- ☐ Muscle cramps
- ☐ Eyebrows are thin or fall out
- ☐ Confusion
- ☐ Increased or irregular menstrual flow

Is it any wonder women struggle so deeply with symptoms when our bodies are going through the natural journey of menopause?

However, those same symptoms may be an indicator of a much deeper imbalance, an autoimmune disorder such as hypothyroidism. All of these may be linked to multiple hormone changes, but the good news is they are extremely treatable with the proper mix of natural supplements alone or in combination with Synthroid, if required. Synthroid alone is rarely the answer, and often the correct mix of herbs may eliminate the need for Synthroid.

Blood tests are essential to diagnose thyroid conditions by measuring the amount of thyroid hormone and thyroid-stimulating hormones in your blood. A full thyroid panel is your best choice: (however frustratingly your doctor may not participate!)

➢ TSH,

➢ free T3 (Triiodothyronine),

➢ free T4 (Thyroxine), and

➢ reverse T3.

So, if this is where you find yourself, what is your best course of action?

The goal of treatment is to return your thyroid back to normal. From an integrative perspective there are a few pillars to this type of treatment. Due to lack of knowledge most women will start with medical treatment and a prescription for hypothyroidism, most commonly Synthroid. This should be followed by more blood tests to ensure your dosage is correct and the medication is working. Your doctor will probably indicate this will be your stand-by medicine for the rest of your life. In my experience, this is not always the case.

I have treated many clients on Synthroid in combination with herbs very successfully. Treating the thyroid alone has the potential for minimal success and will throw off your entire hormone cascade. It is why many women are often frustrated at their lack of success with

Synthroid, anticipating weight loss and other benefits which may rarely occur.

An Integrative Plan for hypothyroidism, on the other hand, would include the following:

Step #1: A Support System for the Thyroid:

This may be a prescription medication of Desiccated Thyroid that is much more effective than Synthroid. Often compounded, this medication is a mix of T3 and T4 from a bovine source (not a synthetic source like Synthroid). Or an alternative and best choice is a therapeutic mix of herbs to target the Thyroid, NO medication.

Step #2: A Customized Mix of Herbal Supplements:

This mix is based on the template of saliva hormone test, symptoms, and medical history. This customized program will provide a foundation of support for other hormones directly and indirectly affecting the thyroid: DHEA, Cortisol, Estradiol, Progesterone, Testosterone (optional). This tailored solution is best developed in combination with the saliva hormone test results and a personal health assessment.

Step #1 and Step #2 should always be combined for optimum results. Thyroid support alone is never the answer.

An integrative approach would also include:

➤ Lifestyle Modification: clean eating, good hydration, moderate exercise;

➤ Weight Loss Program as required, specific to women in menopause;

➤ Morning structure and self-care.

Why are menopausal women exposed to such high risk of thyroid disease?

Aging: Unfortunately, as we age the thyroid starts to slow, and is less able to function at its optimum without any foundational support. Obviously, this is also affected by each woman's lifestyle, fitness level, overall general health, and medical history. Long-term use of Synthroid will negatively impact the functioning of the thyroid, slowing it to a halt as the body becomes dependent on the drug. In a similar fashion, birth control will lower our natural levels of estradiol and progesterone.

Stress: Women are overwhelmed with commitments both in their work and at home to support and 'be it all' for the family. Working full-time and running the day-to-day tasks of a household can be depleting, let alone all the birthday and holiday functions.

I still remember the enjoyable yet sometimes overwhelming duties of four children I was responsible for, plus running a business. As discussed in prior chapters, adrenal fatigue often becomes a factor as the body over produces cortisol to overcome emotional and physical stress. Of course, our environment plays a role (such as, do we have a supportive partner?). As our adrenal glands become a priority in menopause, the building blocks required for thyroid hormones become depleted. If stress becomes chronic it may also cause an imbalance in the estradiol-progesterone axis, causing further degrees of unwanted symptoms.

Estrogen Dominance: Prior to and during menopause, as hormone levels shift, women can easily become estrogen dominant even with low estrogen levels. High estrogen in relation to progesterone can block the thyroid hormone's ability to bind to receptors putting women in a cellular state of functional hypothyroidism. Symptoms vary, but it is often characterized by heavy and irregular cycles. The issue is the similarity between estrogen and thyroid hormone. In a state of estrogen dominance, estrogen can bind to thyroid receptors. Take note that for some women, taking estrogen for menopausal symptoms will only serve to decrease the functionality of the thyroid hormone and can unknowingly put their health at risk.

Progesterone: Another dilemma is also created as progesterone levels drop during menopause, affecting our body's ability to bind T3 (our active thyroid hormone) to its receptors.

Hormone Cascade: The cascade is a series of successive reactions leading to the production of other hormones along the chain. Imbalances in the thyroid will disrupt this pathway. It all starts with cholesterol as the top building block for hormones. Cholesterol supplies our body with the resources to make hormones. Perhaps this explains why men and women develop high cholesterol in their 50s (in addition to the quality of their lifestyle and nutrition).

Unfortunately, due to the over-prescribing of Statins (cholesterol lowering medication), doctors are interfering at times with our bodies' ability to maintain an adequate supply of hormones. Any disruption in the supply of thyroid hormone will disrupt the sequence of events leading possibly to a limited supply of DHEA right down the line to estradiol, progesterone, and testosterone. However, due to their medical history, some patients may not have a choice but to accept the use of the Statins.

However, nothing in our body works independently of each other. It's strongly based on a bio feedback mechanism. That is, our hormones like to feed off each other in a constant quest for balance.

So, What Are Your Next Steps?

As a woman and expert, I always strongly encourage women to have proper testing and consider a customized program of natural supplements to support their hormone cascade from all aspects, either alone or in combination with thyroid medication if required. This is your best choice to support your health, take control back and live the life you so desire.

In addition, as you resolve your symptoms and boost your self-esteem, consider working towards that weight loss goal and shift in body-image you crave if that is still sitting on the back burner of your self-care goals. Get back into your closet of beautiful clothes with a euphoria of renewed self-esteem! *Just remember weight loss during menopause requires a unique approach as you will see in the next chapter when you meet Veronica.*

Thyroid Checklist (also see the comprehensive list at the back of the book)

Overactive Thyroid

- ☐ Hair loss
- ☐ Heat intolerance
- ☐ Unexplained weight loss
- ☐ Large lump in the throat (Goiter)
- ☐ Increased bowel movements
- ☐ Insomnia
- ☐ Light or absent periods
- ☐ Muscle weakness
- ☐ Nervousness or jitteriness
- ☐ Bulging eyes or a 'staring gaze'
- ☐ Trembling in the hands
- ☐ Warm, moist skin
- ☐ Breathlessness
- ☐ Fatigue

Underactive Thyroid

- ☐ Chronic fatigue, weakness
- ☐ Metallic taste in the mouth
- ☐ Dry skin and cracking heels
- ☐ Soft, doughy belly
- ☐ Swelling of the eyelids or face (edema)
- ☐ Anemia
- ☐ Anxiety/ nervousness
- ☐ Cold hands & feet, cold intolerance, low body temperature
- ☐ Constipation
- ☐ Depression and irritability
- ☐ Dry, coarse hair
- ☐ Hair loss
- ☐ Large lump in the throat (Goiter)
- ☐ Headaches and dizziness

Sample 3-day Meal Plan for Hypothyroidism

Day 1

Breakfast: Smoothie

2 glasses of water with lemon

Blend a protein shake with 25 to 30 gm of protein powder, water, a handful of strawberries and 1 tsp of flaxseed oil

Fruit: one apple or one pear

Lunch: Roasted Chicken & Sauteed Peppers

Cook 4 oz of boneless chicken breast with ½ cup of chopped onion

Add clove of garlic and 1 tsp of ground cumin

Sauté ½ cup each of sweet red peppers and yellow peppers

Once cooked place on a bed of romaine lettuce or raw spinach

Dinner: Roasted Steak or Chicken with Quinoa

Cook 4 oz of boneless chicken breast or steak in 2 cups of low sodium beef broth

Add 3 stalks of celery and one small yellow onion

Chopped carrots optional

½ cup of cooked pasta, brown rice, or quinoa

Day 2

Breakfast: Spinach Omelette

Drink 2 cups of water with lemon

3 eggs with spinach

Lunch: Chicken Salad

4 oz grilled chicken breast

3 cups of leaf lettuce

½ cup raw almonds

1/3 cup chopped raw sweet red pepper

1 small pear chopped

Grill the chicken, steam on the stove in water or sodium-reduced broth, or roast in the oven.

Place on bed of leaf lettuce with suggested toppings.

Dinner: Grilled Steak Salad

6 oz of rib eye steak, fat removed

3 cups of leaf lettuce, spinach, or romaine (or a mix)

1 cup of chopped celery sticks

2 mandarin oranges

1 cup of strawberries

2 tbsp of balsamic vinegar

½ tsp of extra virgin oil

Roast steak in the oven with seasonings. Chop on the bed of lettuce with suggested toppings.

Day 3

Breakfast: Pumpkin Smoothie

25 grams/2 tablespoons of canned pumpkin (not pie filling)

2 oz of unsweetened almond milk

30 grams of protein powder

1 ½ tsp of flaxseed oil

½ tsp of ground cinnamon

½ tsp of ground nutmeg

Add water to achieve the texture you want

Lunch: Mexican Bean Salad

4 oz grilled boneless chicken breast

½ cup of lettuce

½ cup of black beans

2 tbsp of sliced raw avocado

3 tsp of shredded mozzarella or feta cheese

Salsa and sour cream (optional! Use in moderation)

Dinner: Herb Roasted Lemon Chicken or White Fish

4-6 oz of boneless skinless chicken breast or white fish

½ lemon

Seasoning of choice

1 small baked sweet potato with skin

Side salad: lettuce, ½ cup cucumber, 1 sliced tomato, 1 tsp olive oil, 1 tbsp balsamic vinegar

Marinate chicken or fish the night before and roast in the oven with sweet potatoes

Releasing Hormonal Weight: Not So Easy

During menopause our body starts to gain weight differently and, at times, dramatically. Women can easily gain 10 pounds in a month, a size, as their hormones shift, and their metabolism slows. Old solutions don't work as our body chemistry has changed and there are more pieces to the puzzle. Solutions need to be tailored and specific to menopause.

As we transition through menopause and our body shape shifts, weight release can become an uphill battle, plagued with frustration and setbacks. After months of disappointment, we may finally recognize that whatever worked in the past is no longer effective due to our new body chemistry. My weight loss journey began at 49 years old, facing the death of a marriage and impending divorce.

At that time, I was also very unhappy with my body image; for me it felt like it happened overnight. I think, however, I was just very distracted with life's responsibilities. I was not paying attention and my self-care had slid to the bottom of my priority list. Like many women in menopause, I had never struggled with my weight, yet confidence was becoming an issue and I often avoided social engagements out of embarrassment.

All around the same time frame, I had ironically started a weight loss service at my integrative clinic specialized and catered to the needs of women my age struggling with menopausal weight gain. Like all the services I offered, I decided to 'take my own medicine' and jump on board both for myself and to better serve my clients in providing clarity and understanding on the new service.

The program was first introduced to me by a fellow colleague; however, at that time the program incorporated a prescription injection which I was not comfortable with out of concern for the side effects. Once I was able to access a homeopathic version, my journey began with confidence.

The program was straightforward, combining clean eating with the natural weight loss formula to burn fat and reset the metabolism. From a scientific perspective it made sense but, as I look back, I recognize I really had no idea what was truly involved when it came to successfully supporting clients' ability to not only release weight to also transition to a healthy sustainable lifestyle. There were some other unknown pieces.

Offering the service seemed simple, yet I wasn't your typical weight loss client. I had no eating disorders or fixations on food. I wasn't a stress eater. The poor habit that was a huge challenge for me was night-time eating. I began on Valentine's Day with no expectations or goals. My weight shifted quickly and after three months I was down 30 pounds and four sizes! My confidence soared and my life shifted dramatically. Soon after, I met my second husband. He swept me off my feet like a princess. I felt young and rejuvenated!

Some of you will identify with this experience, some of you may not. I recognize that our life experiences define the person we are today. The bottom line is weight loss during menopause can be a huge challenge. Understanding all aspects and underlying causes helps put you in the right place both emotionally and intellectually to better set you up for success.

Over the last two years, I began to truly analyze my weight loss system. Looking at clients' failures and successes, I started to integrate new concepts to enhance the program by looking at each client's needs and common challenges. First, during menopause our body starts to gain weight differently and, at times, dramatically. Women can easily gain 10 pounds in a month, a size, as their hormones shift and their metabolism slows. Suddenly our clothes are tight, and our wardrobe becomes limited.

It's no wonder it becomes so disheartening as we look at pictures and compare them to this stranger staring back at us in the mirror.

Losing weight on the program wasn't necessarily difficult. Keeping it off and sustaining a reasonable lifestyle was the challenge. As I started to tell women, "I can get you to the finish line. We need to picture what comes after." Not only does our body gain weight differently during menopause, but our chemistry has also changed, and the puzzle becomes more complicated. Women may exercise and eat properly and often still see no changes on the scale. Old solutions won't work because our hormones have now become a strong influencer on our success. Even exercising seven days a week may not prove to be successful!

I decided the best approach was to complement the saliva hormone kit with the weight release program to target all aspects for women. With my expertise, I realized that part of sustainability and the foundation of the program would be to balance hormones, shift the metabolism and support the thyroid. While I had successfully lost weight, I also had been balancing my hormones prior to menopause which gave my body a better foundation to change.

All our hormones can have the ability to influence our weight; however, Cortisol balance is crucial, which is so often affected by our overwhelming responsibilities as women. Our shoulders are broad, yet our bodies can still take a hit. Too often as I listen to women's stories, I wondered how I could shift their mindset to self-care… another piece of the weight loss puzzle.

Meet Veronica… at 53 years old, having transitioned through surgical menopause in her early 40s, she was the other typical client who had struggled with weight her whole life. We connected immediately during our first phone consultation and began to build a trusting relationship. Her vision was to lose 30 to 50 pounds (as I write this book, she has lost 75!) with the goal of feeling healthy and secure in a new body image. She immediately mentioned how her body had begun to gain weight differently over the last two to three years with the mid-section/belly fat becoming a concern. In addition, one of her bad habits was not feeling hungry and then skipping meals at work. Unfortunately, this slowed her metabolism making it more challenging to release the unwanted weight. Plus, she was eating too much later in the day as opposed to having smaller meals throughout the day.

Asking Veronica how her current body image was affecting her life she said that she always had a healthy self-image, however, that no longer matched the image she saw in the mirror after showering. Her shifting weight made her feel older and unattractive and physically, it was affecting her joints and mobility.

When Veronica jumped on board, I was very transparent. I explained that after 50, the choice of a weight loss program should be very specific to menopause and be sustainable. At our age we do not crave a cookie-cutter program with packaged food and generic supplements. Even calorie counting should be off the table. Our best choice is to eat 'clean' and limit if not eliminate bad carbohydrates to balance blood sugar and reduce hot flashes.

As with all programs, I am a big believer in the support of a natural supplement. In this case it was a homeopathic formula used to burn fat and re-set the metabolism, at a therapeutic dosage that resonates with the client's needs.

If you are researching a suitable weight loss program for menopausal women, I would always consider the following:

1. **Does the program provide a reasonable and sustainable lifestyle?**

2. **Does it provide life coaching to remove old habits that are no longer serving you?**

3. **Is it a long-term solution or a quick fix?**

4. **Does it support our health and encourage self-care?**

5. **Does it incorporate a component to accurately test and balance hormones?**

As Veronica and I worked through her mindset and old habits she began to recognize, like many women, she had a negative emotional attachment to the scale. Together we were able to release this feeling of anxiety by replacing it with confidence that she was moving in the right direction with pride and commitment. She also stopped picking at leftovers during dinner clean-up (absolutely one of my old habits when I was cooking for four children!).

What impressed me with Veronica's journey is she committed step by step to all aspects of the program including self-care. Meditation and movement became a morning routine, the timing of which can be challenging for women with our overwhelming commitments.

As our time together was coming to an end Veronica's goals had far exceeded her expectations as she approached her 'high school' weight. We have remained friends. How could we not after meeting twice a week for over a year!

The greatest compliment and validation: Veronica's self-care continued into a sustainable lifestyle of renewed health and well-being. As we progress to further chapters you will understand how high cortisol, poor stress management and lack of self-care can take us down unwanted pathways.

Weight Loss Challenges During Menopause

One of women's biggest challenges during menopause is weight gain and an often-dramatic shift in body shape. The struggle can be so frustrating as old solutions don't work and we often just give up. Our self-esteem is affected as we longingly look back at old pictures. We often look at the woman in the mirror feeling so disheartened. Who is she? Now is the time to take back control and be accountable to our health. Start now with your own self-analysis of your personal weight loss challenges. Remember, there are four pillars for successful weight release during menopause and all four need to be aligned!!

Losing weight is not a race to the finish line. Living healthy is a choice, not deprivation.

Bad Habits

Part of our weight loss challenge is substituting bad habits that are not serving us, such as stress eating, late dinners, snacking at night and a diet high in bad carbohydrates.

What are your bad habits? (Be honest and transparent with yourself)

_____

_____

_____

_____

Sustainable Lifestyle

Creating a sustainable lifestyle is key to maintaining a successful weight loss for both our health and self-image.

One suggestion is to permanently remove bigger clothing from the closet during a weight-loss journey with the intention of never going back. Substituting milk for cream in your coffee is a small change that makes a big difference over time.

Eliminating the temptations of the drive-thru is a goal to support your healthier lifestyle. Walking a minimum of 15 minutes a day, building up to 45 minutes as desired would be another.

Committing to meal planning and packing a lunch every day instead of buying it is a good example of a change of both lifestyle and eating. For women it's all about being organized. Even a seemingly healthy choice of pre-prepped meals can be high in sodium with unwanted additives. Clean eating should translate to cooking at home!

What are your long-term goals for a sustainable lifestyle?

_____

_____

_____

_____

_____

_____

_____

_____

_____

_____

_____

Hormone Imbalance

The biggest challenge during menopause is that our body starts to gain weight differently and somewhat rapidly as another 10 lbs. magically appear. Often women develop the dreaded 'Muffin Top' around their midsection or carry weight low on their hips and thighs. The reason is that their chemistry has changed and what is going on below the surface has shifted. Their hormones are out of balance and need to be supported. Shifting lifestyle is of great benefit, but hormones are also a dramatic influencer on our weight.

Do you recognize that hormones are affecting your weight and body shape?

_____

_____

_____

_____

_____

_____

_____

What are your symptoms of hormone imbalance?

_____

_____

_____

_____

_____

_____

_____

Slow Metabolism and Thyroid Imbalance

If our hormones are shifting, then our thyroid balance is shifting also. Unfortunately, your blood work may not show the proof. Yet it may become obvious that our metabolism has slowed. It will take a dramatic shift in lifestyle for our body to listen and for the unwanted pounds to shed. Even exercising seven days a week just may not work! In menopause we need to follow a system that will speed up our metabolism to a degree and support the thyroid for us to embrace the longevity of our successful weight loss.

Do you recognize that your metabolism has slowed?

_____

_____

_____

_____

_____

_____

_____

Are you taking natural supplements to support your Thyroid balance? Have you noticed any changes?

_____

_____

_____

_____

_____

_____

_____

Old Solutions Don't Work

As we age and our body starts to gain weight in different areas (think of going from an hourglass to a pear or from an 'average' silhouette to an apple), old solutions may not work or may work to a very limited degree. While exercise is of great value, alone it often won't provide us with the desired results. What worked in the past is no longer serving us as our body chemistry has changed and our weight loss solutions need to be very targeted to our menopause journey.

What weight loss solutions/plans have you tried in the past?

_____

_____

_____

_____

_____

_____

_____

_____

What worked?

_____

_____

_____

_____

_____

_____

_____

_____

The Dangers of High Cortisol

When your internal alarm system is overtaxed by a persistent state of stress and release of cortisol, you may be in a condition of Adrenal Fatigue; you can no longer produce levels of cortisol necessary for optimal body function. Mindfulness is key to managing cortisol levels, as well as keeping ourselves in a healthy environment. Be aware and take control or the journey will become overwhelming.

Managing cortisol and the stress of our environment is one of the pillars of good health. Not always an easy task if we are living in a pool of anxiety and distress.

Cortisol is often called the 'stress hormone' because of its connection to the stress/danger response. However, cortisol is much more than just a hormone released during stress. Understanding cortisol and its effect on the body will help you take action to balance your hormones and achieve good health. When our body is in a constant state of stress our other hormones will be negatively affected as our adrenal glands work to produce excess cortisol during this time of need.

What Does Cortisol Do?

Because most bodily cells have cortisol receptors, it affects many different functions in the body. Cortisol can help control blood sugar levels, regulate metabolism, help reduce inflammation, and assist with memory formulation. It has a controlling effect on salt and water balance and helps control blood pressure. In pregnant women, cortisol also supports the developing fetus during pregnancy. All these functions make cortisol a crucial hormone to protect overall health and well-being.

High cortisol levels can also contribute to changes in a woman's libido and menstrual cycle, even without the presence of Cushing Disease. Anxiety and depression are often linked to high cortisol levels. Supporting our body during these times with natural stress adaptogens (herbal supplements) can prove to be successful; however, it isn't the entire picture.

This hormone also controls the sleep/wake cycle. It is released during times of stress to help your body get an energy boost and better handle an emergency. High cortisol can affect our sleep, weight, anxiety, and clarity of thought. Women in menopause often relate high cortisol to their horrific muffin top (stress fat).

Cortisol is the main hormone released during stress and the fight-or-flight response. This is a natural and protective response to a perceived threat or danger (imagine running from a wild beast or manoeuvring to avoid a collision). Increased levels of cortisol result in a burst of new energy and strength.

In the fight-or-flight response, cortisol suppresses any functions that are unnecessary or detrimental to that response. During a fight-or-flight response, you can have:

- ☐ a rapid heart rate
- ☐ dry mouth
- ☐ stomach upset
- ☐ diarrhea
- ☐ panic

Cortisol release also:

- ☐ suppresses your growth processes
- ☐ suppresses your digestive system
- ☐ suppresses your reproductive system
- ☐ changes how your immune system responds

The Effects of High Cortisol Levels

Over the last 20 years, studies have increasingly revealed that moderate to high cortisol levels may lead to an array of health issues, such as:

Chronic disease. Long-term increased cortisol may increase your risk for high blood pressure, heart disease, Type-2 diabetes, osteoporosis, and other chronic diseases.

Weight gain. Cortisol may increase appetite and signal the body to shift metabolism to store fat.

Lack of energy/difficulty sleeping. It can interfere with sleep hormones which may impact sleep quality and length.

Difficulty concentrating. Also referred to as 'brain fog', some people report trouble focusing and lack of mental clarity.

Impaired immune system. Increased cortisol can hamper the immune system, making it more difficult to fight infections.

Elevated cortisol levels can be caused from many underlying issues such as overactivity or cancer of the pituitary or adrenal glands, chronic stress, and medication side effects.

Further, existing chronic disease (e.g., obesity) may lead to higher cortisol levels, causing a 'chicken or egg' type of scenario.

The Effects of Low Cortisol Levels

On the other side of the equation, you may be producing too little cortisol, or your cortisol may be depleted due to excessive, long-term stress. In extreme cases if your body doesn't make enough cortisol, you may be diagnosed with a condition called Addison's Disease; this is a rare condition requiring care by a specialist hormone doctor called an endocrinologist. Without treatment, this is a potentially life-threatening condition.

Too little cortisol may be due to an imbalance in the pituitary gland or the adrenal gland. The onset of symptoms is often very gradual and therefore easy to dismiss. Symptoms may include fatigue, dizziness (especially when you stand up), loss of appetite and weight loss, muscle weakness that gets worse over time, mood changes, darkening of the skin especially in folds and over scars, diarrhea, nausea and vomiting, and low blood pressure.

When your internal alarm system is overtaxed by a persistent state of stress and release of cortisol, you may be in a state of Adrenal Fatigue; you can no longer produce levels of cortisol necessary for optimal body function.

Therefore, it's best to work with a qualified health professional or integrative practitioner to establish the root cause of your health issues. Along with this, you may want to introduce some effective lifestyle habits that may help you better manage your cortisol levels. As you will see in further chapters, living in an environment of consistent high stress can have a dramatic effect on your health.

The answer you should seek before considering any treatment plan is - Is your cortisol high or low? Remember, high stress can also deplete cortisol over time giving us similar symptoms. The secret for success in any menopausal treatment is proper testing to clearly define your chemistry.

Cortisol Checklist

If you are experiencing:

- ☐ Hair loss
- ☐ High blood pressure
- ☐ High insulin
- ☐ Insulin resistance (diabetes)
- ☐ Irritability
- ☐ Anxiety

- ☐ Low DHEA
- ☐ Low progesterone levels
- ☐ Low libido (sex drive)
- ☐ Low thyroid
- ☐ Mood swings
- ☐ Depression
- ☐ Osteoporosis
- ☐ Poor immune function
- ☐ Weight gain
- ☐ 'Wired but tired' feeling

… you may have excess cortisol.

If you are experiencing:

- ☐ Allergies
- ☐ A burned-out feeling
- ☐ Difficulty handling stress
- ☐ A feeling that you are dragging yourself through every day
- ☐ Increased infections
- ☐ Low blood pressure
- ☐ Waking up tired
- ☐ Muscle stiffness
- ☐ No sex drive (libido)
- ☐ Sensitivity to cold

… you may have low cortisol.

Mindfulness-Based Stress Reduction

Paying attention and being aware of stressful thoughts may help you reduce them. Mindfulness based stress reduction is a strategy that involves becoming more self-aware of stress-provoking thoughts, accepting them without judgement or resistance, and allowing yourself the ability to process them. It also means "re-programming" and releasing old habits that don't serve us.

Training yourself to be aware of your thoughts, breathing, heart rate, and other signs of tension helps you recognize stress when it begins.

By focusing on awareness of your mental and physical state, you can become an objective observer of your stressful thoughts, instead of a victim of them.

Recognizing stressful thoughts allows you to formulate a conscious and deliberate reaction to them. For example, a study involving 43 women in a mindfulness-based program showed the ability to describe and articulate stress was linked to a lower cortisol response.

Stress Reduction should be a central part of our Integrative Plan as it is linked to all aspects of our health. Be prepared in the second half of the book to develop your own integrative plan, take control back and manifest your future!

The Complexity of Estrogen Dominance

Assumptions can often lead us down a dangerous pathway. Be aware that Estrogen Dominance can run rampant during menopause. The question remains: Are our bodies deficient in estrogen or excessive in estrogen with little or no progesterone to balance its effects in the body? Recognize it can be affected by so many factors beyond our control including exposure to xenoestrogens and the toxicity of our personal environment. Check the list and see if the shoe fits… perhaps it is time to be tested!

As stated in earlier chapters, estrogen dominance can have a very profound effect on women's health prior to and during menopause. At times we are so unaware that our actions and assumptions can create somewhat of a health risk. For example, we may increase soya products and supplements to boost estrogen and offset hot flashes assuming we have 'no estrogen' without testing.

Estrogen dominance is a term that describes a condition where a woman can have deficient, normal or excessive estrogen, but have little or no progesterone to balance its effects in the body. Even a woman with low estrogen levels can have estrogen dominance symptoms if she doesn't have enough progesterone.

Excess estrogen causing estrogen dominance is also received trans dermally (through the skin) from all sorts of external sources. These are called Xenoestrogens. These are fat-soluble and non-biodegradable in nature. The major sources of these Xenoestrogens are pesticides, detergents, petroleum products, plastic products, cosmetics, even spermicides used for birth control in diaphragm jellies, condoms and in vaginal gels.

So, think twice when you drink your hot coffee or tea in that plastic or styrofoam cup from your favourite coffee shop. Whatever you do, DO NOT heat your food in plastic cookware. Even best to consider NO microwave at all!

All of these may contribute to estrogen dominance as we head into menopause. I personally removed the microwave from our home over 25 years ago, never to be replaced.

As you will see, the list of symptoms associated with Estrogen Dominance is extensive and I am sure you will connect with at least 2 or 3. The symptoms are:

- ☐ Acceleration of the aging process
- ☐ Allergies, including asthma, hives, rashes, sinus congestion
- ☐ Autoimmune disorders such as lupus erythematosus, thyroiditis, and Sjogren's
- ☐ Breast cancer
- ☐ Breast tenderness
- ☐ Cervical dysplasia
- ☐ Cold hands and feet as a symptom of thyroid dysfunction
- ☐ Decreased sex drive
- ☐ Depression with anxiety or agitation
- ☐ Dry eyes
- ☐ Early onset of menstruation
- ☐ Endometrial (uterine) cancer
- ☐ Fat gain, especially around the abdomen, hips and thighs
- ☐ Fatigue
- ☐ Fibrocystic breasts
- ☐ Foggy thinking
- ☐ Gallbladder disease
- ☐ Hair loss

- ☐ Headaches
- ☐ Hypoglycemia
- ☐ Increased blood clotting (increasing risk of strokes)
- ☐ Infertility
- ☐ Irregular menstrual periods
- ☐ Irritability
- ☐ Insomnia
- ☐ Magnesium deficiency
- ☐ Memory loss
- ☐ Mood swings
- ☐ Osteoporosis
- ☐ Polycystic ovaries
- ☐ Premenopausal bone loss
- ☐ PMS
- ☐ Sluggish metabolism
- ☐ Thyroid dysfunction mimicking hypothyroidism
- ☐ Uterine cancer
- ☐ Uterine fibroids
- ☐ Water retention & bloating
- ☐ Zinc deficiency

When Estrogen Dominance occurs within the body these are some of the results:

- ☐ Endometriosis
- ☐ Blood clots
- ☐ Elevated blood pressure
- ☐ Fibroid breasts
- ☐ Infertility

- [ ] Irregular menstrual flow
- [ ] Uterine fibroids
- [ ] Breast tenderness
- [ ] Mood swings
- [ ] Uterine cancer risk
- [ ] Hair loss
- [ ] Depression
- [ ] Weight gain
- [ ] Migraine headaches
- [ ] Spotting
- [ ] Breast cancer risk
- [ ] Insomnia
- [ ] Inflammation
- [ ] Abnormal pap smears
- [ ] Fluid retention
- [ ] Cramping
- [ ] Vaginal dryness
- [ ] Thyroid imbalances
- [ ] Decrease in memory
- [ ] Low or no sex drive

Strictly speaking, it's possible that we are all - men, women, and children - suffering a little from Estrogen Dominance, because there is so much of it in our environment. You would have to virtually live in a bubble to escape the excess estrogens we're exposed to through pesticides, plastics, industrial waste products, car exhaust, meat, soaps and much of the carpeting, furniture, and paneling that we live with indoors every day.

You may have on-and-off sinus problems, headaches, dry eyes, asthma or cold hands and feet for example, and not know to attribute them to your exposure to Xenohormones. Over time the exposure will cause more chronic problems such as arthritis and premenopausal symptoms and may be a direct or indirect cause of cancer.

The question is how do we avoid it? Estrogen dominance can be reduced by limiting your exposure to environmental toxins or Xenohormones. However, we have little to no control on exposure to some degree, not even knowing the extent of what may be contained in our food. Hence our best choice is to eat as clean as possible.

As you will see in the next chapter, combining estrogen dominance with a stressful environment may not lead to a positive outcome.

My Brief Encounter
With Breast Cancer

In July 2021, I found my life thrown in a very unexpected direction. Self-care had always been a priority, yet my tool kit was depleted, and I was finding myself in a constant state of distress. Surrounded by an environment of negativity, I struggled to pull myself out of this deep hole. This was my end result... a gift.

I am sitting in what I call 'the reading room' writing the next chapter of my book. The first draft of the book was to be completed by September 6th, yet it is already the 18th. Reality has thrown me off track and into a very different direction than I had ever anticipated. Yet as I look back, I should have clearly seen this coming. Now I recognize some of the signs: increased fatigue (blamed it on the new puppy!), discomfort along the bra line (doctor said it was indigestion!), and a sudden weight loss of 20 lbs I didn't even notice!

For over two years I was drowning in a deep pool of personal stress that I couldn't free myself from. Yet here I was, a life coach and women's health expert teaching my clients about the importance of self-care and a positive mind-set. I had all those tools in place; however, they had become severely depleted and off balance no matter how I tried to pull myself out of this deep hole.

I thought I was doing okay; however, I truly wasn't. Living within this environment of constant discomfort, I just couldn't set myself free no matter how hard I tried to succeed. Perhaps doing better than most would, yet definitely not winning the race. My thoughts and my environment were attracting illness and I felt so out of control. Everything big and small sent my mind reeling. My anxiety was constantly peaked. No matter how well I ate, how much I exercised and how many supplements I took, my stress was overtaking my life.

Yet within this debacle I actually did not feel unhappy because I always had the outlet and passion of my work supporting women in their journey through menopause. However, by not making changes to my personal environment, I was avoiding part of my own self-care. Doing all the right things from eating to exercise did not make me untouchable from disease or illness.

So, when I was surprisingly …or not so surprisingly… diagnosed with breast cancer in July 2021, I actually felt the universe had given me a gift. A gift to make corrections and set boundaries to those around me. A gift to establish what was truly important. A gift to embrace the simple, quiet, peaceful life I was desperately seeking. An event that happened FOR me, not TO me.

Perhaps I didn't need to work so hard and be the over-achiever. Perhaps I already had everything I needed in my life. Now I was finding inner peace. The gift I received kindly and quickly released my anger and resentment to those around me. I was not scared. I felt re-born. Yet I also had to be accountable to this challenge as I had not been responding to the unwanted events in my life appropriately, allowing behaviour within my close circle that was not in alignment with what I knew was healthy. Definitely not aligned with my beliefs and inner spirituality. Certainly not aligned with my personal perception of the world as positive place, always believing in the good, & fairness of humanity.

However strong I was to meet this head on, there was also a streak of stubbornness. I had always told myself that radiation and chemo-therapy would never be an option. Even though I was a pharmacist, I was also a strong advocate and leader in natural, integrative medicine. I had spent the last 25 years plus taking supplements and at 58 was on zero medication.

My stubborn streak persisted when I met my team of doctors. Perhaps I was scared as I quickly became angry and arrogant with the radiologist. I finally had to silence myself and listen. After all, I needed all the resources to make the right decisions for myself. It was not only the doctor's expertise and my own perception that guided me. I had two guardian angels watching over me. Sandra, a client, and breast cancer survivor, and Jennifer, my pre-op nurse. Both of whom shared their knowledge and personal experiences with breast cancer to lead me along the best pathway.

Prior to surgery my next hurdle was telling the children. At first, I wanted nothing more but to be silent, not wanting to give my diagnosis too much real estate in my mind. I truly felt the less I shared my news, the better I would be able to heal. I decided not to tell my youngest as it was a week away from his 19th birthday. I set up a zoom meeting with the older three and quietly revealed my challenge. Even saying the "C" word aloud was difficult, perhaps as it made my circumstance real. I also felt that the world treated the 'C' word with doom and gloom.

As I told my children, many, many people survive cancer, and I would be no different.

I started to listen to Wayne Dyer with so much conviction, building a strong relationship together with my new tablet. Every morning I would repeat the following affirmations: "I am healthy, I am well, I am cancer-free. And this, too, shall pass!"

When I told my hairdresser and friend I had the 'C' word, she cried. "Why would you come into the shop with Covid?" I said, "No, the other 'C' word," and we both laughed.

Confident that I could face a lumpectomy and radiation, my surgery was booked. Yet the MRI did not read well. Two days prior to my surgery, Sandra suggested I talk to my surgeon. I reached out to him, and our conversation was very transparent. The MRI suggested a lot of calcifications (pre-cancerous cells) plus multi-focal invasion. He was not confident that one surgery would be enough to remove all the problem areas. His best recommendation was a single mastectomy. The decision was in my hands.

I got off the phone in tears. After all, I was still attempting to adjust to the 'C' word and lumpectomy. Suddenly I was heading in a totally different direction. The next morning, I e-mailed the doctor, agreeing with his recommendation. Twenty-four hours prior to surgery I committed to the mastectomy with fear and anxiety.

My life had changed so quickly and dramatically, I had very little to no time for acceptance. While registering in pre-op, I broke down in tears to my nurse, Jennifer, telling her I was unsure of my decision to have a single mastectomy. She held my hand like an angel and shared her story of surviving breast cancer. She assured me that the mastectomy was my best chance to walk out of the hospital cancer-free.

"Today," she said, "you will leave cancer-free. With a multitude of time to spend with your children." The surgeon kindly told me I could cancel the surgery if I wasn't ready. Yet I felt trapped with no choice but to follow through with my decision. I woke up in post-op in a panic, anxious and scared. Had I made the right decision? Ten days after surgery when I received the pathology report, it was clear. I had made the absolute best decision. My margins were clear as well as my lymph nodes. I was extremely lucky to be Stage 1. My positive affirmations had worked.

I had always told my clients I believed we could heal our body with our mind. Perhaps I should have kept those thoughts to myself. Now due to the law of attraction, the universe was strongly testing my theory. I continued to heal my body with my renewed mind-set and the mellowing of my soul in addition to eating organic and juicing daily!

As my healing began, so did my acceptance of my current situation. One of the challenges I saw for cancer patients is it starts to feel like a race. The cancer versus me. You attempt not to be overly consumed with eating properly and taking as many supplements as possible. Such a small price to pay for longevity.

Luckily, I was fairly on track, yet there is always room for improvements. Even small changes can produce huge adjustments in our health. From a nutritional perspective it meant buying organic, juicing daily, and doubling up on my current supplement regime. The biggest lifestyle improvement for me was choosing to be alone in a positive environment that would facilitate and nurture my healing. Being strong enough to release those relationships that were no longer serving me.

At the beginning of this story when I first visited my family doctor he said, "I bet you a coffee the lumps are benign." I later told him with humour he owed me a five-dollar Starbucks. Once I saw the concerned look on the radiologist's face during the biopsy, I knew my life was going to shift dramatically. I think the biggest shock during the biopsy was wondering how I had allowed myself to enter this place of illness. Could this be happening to *me*? How had this become my story?

Lying in the hospital bed I asked myself, "How did I end up here?" As I stated to my young oncologist, "You don't understand… I exercise five times per week and eat a lot of kale." He smiled and remarked, "Well, keep doing it!"

Sadly, he also reminded me that all women my age have a 1 in 5 risk factor for breast cancer. He also told me my cancer was estrogen positive, which was a good diagnosis, yet unfortunately also opened the door for a 5-year treatment plan of chemo, if required. As my risk of re-occurrence was 6% (single digits!) I kindly made an informed decision to refuse his recommendation for chemotherapy.

In the end I don't know if I ever would have accepted it. Perhaps I would have found a natural treatment centre somewhere in the Caribbean. However, my message is this: I was a slim, healthy woman on zero medications who was estrogen dominant. Obviously, it's always extremely difficult to control our environment and reduce our stress even with all our tools in place.

Acknowledging my circumstance for me was never about playing the blame game. I looked at this challenge as an opportunity to grow and make some corrections in my life. There are no mistakes. Everything happens as it should. I strongly believe the universe brought me this lesson for several reasons. I wasn't aware how much my self-care was falling behind. Plus, I am a teacher; here to teach and share my life experiences with women in my circle.

Four months post-op and I have healed well with no chemo and no radiation. A gift! Though my weight and energy dipped I never felt or looked sick; it was just a predicament and a life-altering experience. I know that isn't the case for everyone.

Acceptance also meant recognizing the necessity to make solid adjustments to my heart and soul. My perspective on life shifted immediately. Perhaps I already had everything I needed: four healthy kids, money in the bank and a community of clients I adored. I started to question my gratitude; was it conscious or sub-conscious?

Every lesson is a platform to teach women the importance of serenity, inner peace, and harmony. Acceptance is surrendering to what is, with the confidence that "everything will work out for me." With relief, it allows us to release our existing struggles, replacing them with our ability to pause and enjoy the quiet.

My message is clear. Are you monitoring the stress of your personal environment?

Are you setting kind boundaries to those closest to you? My risk for breast cancer was extremely low. I was never on Estrogen or HRT. I had no genetic predisposition. I believe my cancer was triggered from the stress of my environment. With rapid intervention, self-care, and an abundance of resilience I quickly travelled the road to wellness because of all the tools I already had in place – plus the shifting of my mind-set. My new emotional state of mind being the biggest part of my cure.

Every day I repeated to myself "I am healthy, I am well, I am cancer-free." My positive mind-set helped overcome this challenge with great resilience to heal my body. "My Brief Encounter With Breast Cancer" is a story of hope! A gift that forced me to take control of my life again!

Committing to Self-Care

Balancing our hormones through tailored solutions is an important piece of the menopause journey, yet so is self-care and the health of our personal environment. By educating women on the benefits of self-care and embracing a positive mindset, my own beliefs began to shift recognizing how my thoughts were guiding my destiny in all aspects of life from relationships to health. The first step in self-care is to start your morning with peace and tranquility…

Committing to Self-Care

As a woman with a career and a mother of four children I can relate to why women too often put themselves last. I remember the race I was running as a young mom with a career; family, of course, came first. I certainly don't regret those times. In fact, I miss those early years of motherhood and often wish I could go back in time. At my age, however, I believe there is a paradigm shift where perhaps we can begin to think more of self-care and the importance of a structured morning routine.

Would I have considered it in my 30s and 40s? Absolutely not. However, I also had little experience with how self-care would impact my life and those around me. Although uncomfortable in the beginning stages, I began to recognize that it was not only self-respectful to put myself first, at times it can become a means of survival. Self-care supports our ability to release unwanted stress and anxiety which can put our health and immune system at risk.

Self-care is a huge commitment with many far-reaching benefits, yet it also takes patience, diligence, commitment, and learning. In the beginning of my career self-care was never spoken of and perhaps I also was too 'medical' in my approach. My goal was to resolve the clients' symptoms. It took years of learning to strongly recognize the connection between the mind, body, and illness, knowing how our mind can truly heal our body or, conversely, create illness.

As I grew in my expertise and through my own life challenges, I started to incorporate life coaching in my practice, educating women on the benefits of self-care and embracing a positive mind-set. My own beliefs began to shift recognizing how my thoughts were guiding my destiny in all aspects of life from relationships to health. Adopting the realization that "What you think about you bring about", creating and manifesting my future through thought alone became a focus. I realized how powerful only 15 minutes of meditation in the morning could be to re-direct my day.

If I could speak to my younger self, I would have done it years ago instead of running a race as soon as my feet hit the floor, being distracted by the digital world and a host of responsibilities.

As I became older and wiser, I realized that I could create my future by thoughts alone as my mind truly didn't know the difference between the present and the future.

Balancing our hormones through tailored solutions is an important piece of the menopausal journey, yet so is self-care and the health of our personal environment. Your circle of influence, that is, the first five people surrounding you, creates that environment.

My self-care journey began by recognizing the tranquility of the 5am morning when the world is quiet. Instead of jumping on my computer, I started my day with a cup of coffee sitting on the sofa and looking out the window, clearing my mind and prioritizing my day. Certainly, a very soulful gesture for my morning cortisol levels. From there my morning routine grew to embrace meditation, journaling, reading and movement. I recognized that even 15 minutes of meditation alone provided more clarity, less brain fog, and increased my productivity throughout the day.

As I began to nurture my clients with this model the strength, depth, and value of those trusting relationships grew.

Meet Sandra, a beautiful woman with a sordid past of many health challenges including breast cancer. As I moved my business online, I began to reach a much broader audience of women such as Sandra, who I knew were desperately seeking answers, frustrated at times with traditional medicine.

I gravitated to Sandra's aura. She had a glow she didn't recognize, and we connected immediately. I felt the passion to serve her to the best of my abilities as many practitioners had rarely met her health needs and expectations. Like many women Sandra was all consumed with work and the responsibilities at home. Her health was deeply challenged, yet she refused to put herself first, even after her diagnosis of breast cancer.

Sandra's family history of breast and ovarian cancer was extensive and heart-breaking. Sadly, her maternal ancestors carried the BRCA1 mutation.

By 2014, Sandra made a wise decision to have an oophorectomy. By then her mother had died of ovarian cancer, multiple aunts of breast cancer and her sister was struggling with both ovarian and breast cancer. At that time, the doctors also recommended a double mastectomy, yet Sandra was scared to commit, feeling her body was already being traumatized by removing all her womanhood.

As surgical menopause hit hard, she chose to use Estradiol and Prometrium (progesterone), not necessarily her best choice based on her history. As the hormone replacement kicked in, she felt euphoric, yet fear always lurked in her sub-conscious mind. Fear took over and she booked her double mastectomy for January 2020, not realizing it would be too late.

After a wonderful family trip to Portugal in July 2019, Sandra was diagnosed with breast cancer. It was a very difficult find as it was small and very deeply imbedded in the chest. If you talked to Sandra today, she would sadly say she would forever regret the decision to hold off on the double mastectomy. Yet at that time it felt like the right decision.

Now she lives one day at a time with acceptance not only of her new body, but also her past decisions.

With my expertise, I wondered why the doctors would recommend hormone replacement with Sandra's history, yet I kept my thoughts to myself. I also understand why women make those decisions. Surgical menopause can be so disruptive and debilitating, affecting our ability to function in all aspects of our life. With no warning or preparation our hormonal support is suddenly removed. Our bodies are plagued with symptoms of raging hot flashes, uncontrolled night sweats, insomnia and more. Our body image and self-esteem shift as our weight often changes.

Sandra did find herself in this position even more so once her hormone treatments were suddenly stopped and post-surgery chemotherapy began. All her menopause symptoms returned with a vengeance and her weight escalated.

Embracing her health outside of traditional medicine required a mentor to guide her. Preferring a women's health expert who had walked in her shoes, we committed to each other. Our mentorship not only needed to support her physically, but also emotionally and spiritually. I kindly explained to Sandra that our emotional and physical health are very interconnected and continuously interact with each other. Could our mind heal our body? As her guide, I led Sandra into the unknown world of Integrative Medicine. Little did I know, Sandra was soon to be my mentor and guide.

As the medical system was no longer serving her, Sandra crossed the threshold with me to Integrative Medicine, adopting a treatment plan with the power of high-grade pharmaceutical supplements, understanding that medicinal hormones were no longer her best choice. Even without her medical history, many women often fear the side effects of HRT, yet at times also crave a better quality of life compared to suffering in silence with multiple unaddressed symptoms of menopause.

Sandra's journey had many ups and downs as she worked diligently to lower her pharmaceutical dosages of a variety of medication. I always emphasized that mind-set would also influence her success as well as her environment, not yet knowing her challenges at home. The withdrawal effect of lowering the dosages of the pharmaceuticals, as her body always anticipated deliverance of the medication, were overwhelming at times.

I encouraged her that I had assisted many, many women in transitioning from the pharmaceutical world to the world of natural medicine with great success; however, everyone's journey varies based on their history, their mindset, and their ability to accept the challenges. I asked her to picture the outcome and not to over worry the process... confident that success was on its way, and she could manifest her desires.

Still, the missing piece for Sandra was self-care. She prided herself as a traditional wife and mother to always take care of the home first, even though her two boys were now young adults. My hope was always that her mindset would shift to pay significantly more attention to her self-care as a means of healing.

As our relationship grew and transitioned from practitioner and client to friends, Sandra shared her reality. She was living in a toxic environment, lonely in an unhappy marriage. I strongly continued to encourage her morning rituals and self-care to buffer her environment. Having worked in natural medicine for decades and worked with hundreds of women (too many sadly in Sandra's position), I knew the strong connection between our environment and our health. Understanding that our environment can create illness, yet our mind could also heal our body. Hence, the power of the positive mindset.

Here was Sandra's Self-Care Checklist:

Note: Digital distraction was to be avoided for the first hour of each morning!

Positive mind-set: Positive thinking creates clarity and reduces stress/cortisol levels. It takes consistency and needs to be worked on daily through gratitude and meditation. Start your day with the following question: "How can I make today a great day?"

My commitment:

_____

_____

_____

_____

Movement: Regular exercise is a great commitment to lower cortisol and increase clarity. Even small efforts produce great benefits to increase energy levels and productivity. Commit to a minimum of 3-5 times per week, even for 20 minutes, and the results will line up quickly.

My commitment:

_____

_____

_____

_____

Meditation: It is surprising what a powerful tool meditation can be to improve sleep. Meditation can not only enhance sleep it also can lower stress levels. Pick a meditation that speaks to you for 5 minutes minimum every morning and evening. Sit quietly to clear your mind. Our best success is to have structure and routine following the 21-day rule for maximum success (as it takes 21 days to change a habit).

My commitment:

_____

_____

_____

_____

Journaling: Another powerful tool to improve our mindset and provide clarity with positive self-talk mixed with gratitude.

My commitment:

_____

_____

_____

_____

Learning: The acquisition of knowledge means growth. Learning can provide simple tools for self-care through quiet reading at times when the world is still sleeping, and our creative juices are heightened. Reading can provide awareness and often clear our mental fog.

My commitment:

_____

_____

_____

_____

Sandra finally committed to creating a consistent morning routine of three success habits with the commitment of a full-time job, seven days a week. For Sandra these morning rituals created structure, increased productivity, and momentum in her life.

Optimizing her morning began to boost her confidence levels and lower cortisol which in turn supported her lagging immune system.

Today, Sandra has turned the corner on self-care and being accountable to #1. Two years post mastectomy she has taken the leap of faith to finally have the strength and confidence to book her re-constructive surgery. On the home front her family has committed to counselling and her environment has become much less toxic. It all began with developing her Integrative Plan.

DEVELOPING YOUR INTEGRATIVE PLAN

What To Do Next?
Develop Your Integrative Plan

There are four main pillars to treating menopause as a whole package for women from nutrition to hormone balance to stress management to motion.

As women it's important to recognize our mind-body connection and how our emotional health is strongly connected to our physical health. In addition, all the pieces to the puzzle need to line up including proper nutrition, moderate exercise, stress management, releasing old habits that no longer serve you, maintaining a positive mindset, creating morning structure, and much more.

Start slowly or jump right in. The choice is yours. Just remember structure and consistency are key. Consider this a full-time job, seven days a week. NO EXCUSES! Part-time commitment produces part-time results. Creating structure, routine and commitment can be uncomfortable in the beginning; however, with discomfort comes growth.

When your body and mind become aligned, you have the willpower to reach your destiny and the energy to move on to your next great task. Set your boundaries and move forward in the name of self-care. Taking good care of ourselves is a choice and creates a very powerful impact to those around us when we take responsibility. It's time to trust and listen to our inner voice. Creating our own enchanted life as we move gracefully through menopause. The final chapter!

The Integrative Check List...A Place to Start

Today is a new day! Commit to yourself and embrace your self-care, your self-love. Start by committing to a structured morning with at least one of these strategies to deliver benefits that you'll be able to feel immediately, and that can make adding more strategies easier. It's all about taking control, making yourself a priority, and creating your own routine of self-care.

☐ **Morning Structure:**

Choose three (3) of the following and commit to 20 minutes of each first thing in the morning. Take time for your self-care, with confidence that it will help to balance your cortisol, give clarity to your day, and increase productivity.

A) journal

B) meditate

C) movement

D) read books

E) reflection

F) plan your day

G) listen to podcasts

H) listen to audio books

Do not participate in digital distraction for the 1st hour - no e-mails, no cell phone, no television. This morning structure is meant to create self-awareness and restore inner peace and tranquility.

Morning structure and how we start our day has a dramatic influence on how it unfolds. Shifting your mindset to Positive is an essential piece.

"How can I make today a great day?"

My Commitment: My Start Date:

1) _____   _____

2) _____   _____

3) _____   _____

☐ Lifestyle Modification:

Take an honest inventory of your current lifestyle. Remember, do not look at this as deprivation. It is a choice to improve your health, release some unwanted weight, and prevent disease state. Even small consistent change could start the journey of releasing unwanted weight and improving self-image.

The more we commit to our self-care, the more we value and love ourselves. Start now to break your old destructive habits and replace with new habits to serve your new rituals of self-care!

My current lifestyle:

Alcohol per day		Daily water consumption (2L minimum)	
Pop per day		Sugar cravings (rate from 1 to 10)	
Caffeine per day		Meal planning	
Consumption of bad carbohydrates		Batch cooking/Food prep	
Snacking at night		Fasting (7pm to 11am)	

☐ **Consistent Exercise: "Movement is Medicine"**

Exercise is a pillar of health with a multitude of benefits, but it doesn't have to be extreme. Many women exercise excessively seven days a week with little to no results in releasing weight. It's best to be realistic and frame your intentions. Exercise provides clarity and lowers cortisol.

As 'motion is lotion' it lubricates our stiff joints. Exercise and building even minimal muscle mass will positively shift our resistant metabolism. It also builds our self-esteem and increases our energy. Even a little exercise will dramatically shift our day.

If you're new to exercise, walking is your best bet. Start with going around the block, then go around twice, or go farther. Wait until the kids are in school or until night fall to embrace the quiet. Even better, find a similarly motivated friend and encourage each other.

Morning exercise will front load our day giving us the energy, confidence, and peacefulness to start our day.

My commitment:

_____

_____

_____

_____

_____

_____

_____

_____

_____

_____

☐ Mind-Set:

Mind-set is central to self-care. At times for women, it seems to come with age and learning to take care of #1. Mind-set is a muscle that needs to be worked daily with awareness. Start in the morning before your feet hit the floor running. Shift your mind-set by deciding "how to make today a great day" and/or what to be grateful for. Remember, it's all linked to the law of attraction and our ability to manifest or create what we want by setting our intentions.

Manifestation means pre-paving the future to what we want. Pre-paved moments could be five years from now, one year from now, 60 days from now, or 24 hours from now. Your sub-conscious mind really doesn't know the difference between the present and the future, so think about things the way you want them to be and prepare for what's to come!

With kindness and generosity, let's choose to take responsibility for ourselves. Learn to listen and nurture our inner voice. Part of our mindset is also setting boundaries to those around us. Finding a place of peace and tranquility, knowing we are on course. Confident to ask the universe for what we want!

Mind-set affects our emotional, spiritual, and physical health. It allows us to heal and prevent disease. It advocates for our Immune System.

Start your day with a positive affirmation. Repeat it throughout the day. If a situation goes sideways out of your control, immediately switch back to positive and remember all you have to be grateful for. Do not let that one negative circumstance derail all your carefully laid plans.

With a positive mind-set comes a clear heart. Our mind-set and heart-set need to be aligned. It means letting go of past hurt, frustration, and disappointments. Otherwise, we are only pretending to lock the intentions of a positive mind-set. Daily gratitude and affirmations are part of this healing.

Remember - happiness is an inside job

Before you fall asleep replay three gratitudes for the day and meditate for five minutes to clear your subconscious mind, your internal hard drive.

A positive mindset can manifest or create our future and the destination we desire.

Daily Affirmations (such as 'I am...', 'I will...', 'I can...'):

_____

_____

3 Things to Be Grateful for:

1) _____

2) _____

3) _____

Next, let's define who you are with awareness and commitment to embracing change. First however, let's be clear on the symptoms you are still struggling with and who you are at this time. Recognizing that nothing changes unless we change!

Hormone Checklists: Finding Your Blueprint!

Symptoms are your body's way of telling you something is off balance. Saliva Testing is the only way to definitively identify baseline hormone levels and create a guided treatment plan. Self-diagnosis is never wise. Tracking your symptoms in preparation for an appointment with your integrative practitioner(s) can frame your discussions with and increase your feeling of being an informed participant, having the ability to advocate for yourself.

An imbalance in one area can have downstream effects and causes imbalances in multiple areas. An integrative approach means identifying the cause of your symptoms rather than just masking them with medication.

Working with the root cause of your symptoms means your treatment plan will help you to feel better in often a short period of time and return you to a state of balance in the long term. Please complete the Hormone Checklist before proceeding to meet "The Girls". Review it each time you move forward to another Case Study, so your symptoms are front of mind and your perception is clear. This will assist your learning very specific to who you are and your ability to identify with the women you are about to meet.

Let's get started!

PROGESTERONE

Low Progesterone

☐ Anxiety

☐ Difficulty managing stress

☐ Elevated cortisol levels

☐ Estrogen dominant conditions such as uterine fibroids, fibrocystic breasts, ovarian cysts, PCOS, breast cancer, thickening of the uterine lining, endometriosis

☐ Headaches

☐ Heavy periods

☐ Low bone density

☐ Recurring miscarriage

☐ Water retention

☐ Weight gain around the abdomen

High/excess Progesterone

☐ Breast swelling and pain

☐ Depression or low mood

☐ Excess facial hair

☐ Feeling sleepy, drowsy

☐ Over production of insulin (hyper insulinemia)

☐ Low libido

☐ Oily skin

ESTROGEN

Low Estrogen

☐ Brain fog

☐ Vaginal dryness

☐ Painful intercourse

☐ Thinning of the vaginal wall (vaginal atrophy)

☐ Recurring urinary tract infections (UTIs)

Excess Estrogen

☐ Adult acne

☐ Anemia

☐ Worsening of asthma

☐ Period problems (irregular, long or short, heavy)

☐ Raging hot flashes and night sweats

☐ Fluid retention

☐ Gallstones

☐ Irritability

☐ Loss of sex drive

☐ Memory loss

☐ Depression

☐ PMS

☐ Weight gain

☐ Estrogen dominant conditions such as uterine fibroids, fibrocystic breasts, ovarian cysts, PCOS, breast cancer, thickening of the uterine lining, endometriosis

TESTOSTERONE

Low Testosterone/ DHEA

☐ Fatigue

☐ High cortisol

☐ Loss of strength and stamina

☐ Low or no sex drive

☐ Memory decline

☐ Muscle wasting and weakness (chin muscles start sagging)

☐ Osteopenia

☐ Osteoporosis

☐ Sleep problems

☐ Vaginal dryness

Excess Testosterone/ DHEA

☐ Acne, oily skin

☐ Facial hair growth

☐ Hair loss

☐ Ovarian cysts and/or polycystic ovarian syndrome (PCOS)

☐ Weight gain

☐ Insulin resistance (pre-diabetes, diabetes)

THYROID

Overactive/ Hyperthyroid

☐ Hair loss

☐ Heat intolerance

☐ Unexplained weight loss

☐ Large lump in the throat (Goiter)

☐ Increased bowel movements

☐ Insomnia

☐ Light or absent periods

☐ Muscle weakness

☐ Nervousness or jitteriness

☐ Bulging eyes or a 'staring gaze'

☐ Trembling in the hands

☐ Warm, moist skin

☐ Breathlessness

☐ Fatigue

THYROID

Low Thyroid/ Hypothyroid

- ☐ Anemia
- ☐ Anxiety/ nervousness
- ☐ Chronic fatigue, weakness
- ☐ Cold hands & feet, cold intolerance, low body temperature
- ☐ Constipation
- ☐ Metallic taste in the mouth
- ☐ Dry skin and cracking heels
- ☐ Depression and irritability
- ☐ Soft, doughy belly
- ☐ Dry, coarse hair
- ☐ Swelling of the eyelids or face (edema)
- ☐ Hair loss
- ☐ Feeling unable to breathe deeply
- ☐ Large lump in the throat (Goiter)
- ☐ High cholesterol
- ☐ Headaches and dizziness
- ☐ Heart palpitations
- ☐ Impaired memory
- ☐ Infertility and/or recurring miscarriage
- ☐ Insomnia
- ☐ Low basal temperature
- ☐ Night sweats
- ☐ Poor concentration

- ☐ Declining vision
- ☐ Difficulty concentrating, racing thoughts
- ☐ Persistent and sometimes severe menopause symptoms that carry on for years
- ☐ Slow pulse
- ☐ Shortness of breath
- ☐ Slow metabolism (indicated by new weight gain, especially around the hips)
- ☐ Sudden change in personality
- ☐ Low T3, T4, or T7
- ☐ High TSH, over 2.0
- ☐ Low progesterone-to-estrogen ratio
- ☐ Hormonal imbalances (indicated by fibroids, ovarian or breast cysts, painful and/or heavy periods, endometriosis, PMS, frequent menstrual cycles)

ADRENAL STRESS

- ☐ Alcohol intolerance
- ☐ Asthma/bronchitis
- ☐ Blurred vision
- ☐ Cold hands, feet
- ☐ Cravings for stimulants like caffeine, sugar, junk food, salt
- ☐ Dizziness upon waking, or when standing up
- ☐ Digestive problems
- ☐ Depression
- ☐ Swelling in the hands and/or feet
- ☐ Excessive perspiration
- ☐ Increased or excessive urination
- ☐ Light sensitivity
- ☐ New food allergies
- ☐ Headaches
- ☐ Heart palpitations
- ☐ High cortisol
- ☐ Hypoglycemia
- ☐ Irritability
- ☐ Insomnia or disrupted sleep (hard to go back to sleep)
- ☐ Inflammation and joint or muscle pain including bursitis and arthritis
- ☐ Knee problems
- ☐ Low back pain
- ☐ Tired feet
- ☐ Nervousness/anxiety

- ☐ Muscle twitches
- ☐ Poor concentration
- ☐ Recurring infections
- ☐ Ulcers
- ☐ Low energy, excessive fatigue after exertion
- ☐ Increase or loss of skin pigment (an indication of the most advanced cases of adrenal exhaustion; skin will look tanned)

CORITSOL

Excess Cortisol

- ☐ Hair loss
- ☐ High blood pressure
- ☐ High insulin
- ☐ Insulin resistance (diabetes)
- ☐ Low progesterone
- ☐ Low sex drive (libido)
- ☐ Low thyroid
- ☐ Mood swings and depression
- ☐ Osteoporosis
- ☐ Poor immune function
- ☐ Weight gain
- ☐ Feeling 'wired but tired'

Low Cortisol

- ☐ Allergies
- ☐ Feeling burned out
- ☐ Difficulty handling stress
- ☐ Sensitivity to cold
- ☐ Increased infections
- ☐ Low blood pressure
- ☐ Waking up tired
- ☐ Muscle stiffness
- ☐ No sex drive
- ☐ Feeling like you are dragging through the day

SYMPTOMS/INDICATORS OF PRE/PERI-MENOPAUSE

- ☐ 35 years or older
- ☐ Lower libido
- ☐ Endometriosis
- ☐ Fibroid breast cysts
- ☐ Thinning hair
- ☐ Headaches
- ☐ Heavy or longer periods, clotting
- ☐ Hot flashes and/or night sweats
- ☐ Insomnia or disrupted sleep
- ☐ Forgetfulness
- ☐ PMS symptoms
- ☐ Adult acne/skin outbreaks
- ☐ A gain of ~10 pounds and a bloated abdomen
- ☐ Uterine fibroids

SYMPTOMS/INDICATORS OF MENOPAUSE

- ☐ 45 years or older
- ☐ No period for 12 consecutive months or longer
- ☐ No desire for sex
- ☐ Feeling anxious, irritable, and easily tired
- ☐ Gaining weight
- ☐ Hot flashes and/or night sweats
- ☐ Painful intercourse
- ☐ Urinary incontinence

☐ Brain fog or memory issues

☐ Insomnia or disrupted sleep

☐ Excessively dry skin and wrinkling

☐ Vaginal dryness

☐ Yeast infections

Saliva Hormone Test Report – for illustration purposes only

Salivary Hormone Results			
		Phase	Reference Range
Estradiol pmol/L	7.5	Follicular	2.8-8.8 pmol/L
		Peak*	4.5-19.1 pmol/L
		Luteal	2.8-8.2 pmol/L
		Menopausal	3.7-9.4 pmol/L
		Male	3.1-7.4 pmol/L
		*Peak = Days 11 and 12	
Testosterone pmol/L	66	Premenopausal	34-148 pmol/L
		Menopausal	34-148 pmol/L
		Male	110-513 pmol/L
Progesterone pmol/L	299	Follicular	17-321 pmol/L
		Peak *	151-829 pmol/L
		Luteal	33-452 pmol/L
		Menopausal	45-370 pmol/L
		Male	31-280 pmol/L
		*Peak = Days 18 and 20	
P/E2 Ratio	27	Follicular	10-85
		Luteal	8-80
		Menopausal	12-62
DHEA 7am-9am	164		71-640 pg/ml

Cortisol Results	7am - 9am*	11am - 1pm*	3pm - 5pm*	10pm - 12am*
Patient Result (mcg/dL)>>	1.052			
Reference Range(mcg/dL) *Based on Collection Times	0.097-0.337			
Actual Collection Time	7:00am			

You may look at this report and say, 'Everything appears to be within the menopausal ranges as outlined, so what's the problem?' From an integrative perspective balance is when your reading lands in the middle of the menopausal range. High and low numbers can cause similar symptoms and need to be treated. Also, the question is: where is your body progressing to? What other symptoms could these results transgress to? This will also define your integrative plan with an eye to prevention.

This is where a women's health expert and integrative practitioner adds value, identifying potential indicators that may call for both preventive measures and more aggressive treatment as required. Guiding the client as a unique individual.

What Are Nutraceuticals?
A Little Science!

As you have learned in previous chapters, through the mentors I met in my life I started to embrace the value of Integrative Medicine and the power of Phytotherapy, or Herbalism. I recognized over the years that hormone balance is a very delicate dance that requires the body to remain very flexible in its ability to sustain the hormone levels required for optimum health. The dance is on-going and affected by many outside forces including our environment, nutrition, and stress levels. It also changes each decade as we journey towards menopause.

If you recall, Maria introduced me to a high grade of herbal supplements which I eventually incorporated into my family, supporting the health of myself and my children, plus my practice of Integrative Medicine. Wellpoint Nutraceuticals are the brand-name supplements I've highlighted in the case studies that you are about to read for the 'girls' you are going to meet.

As I learned, Phytotherapy is the use of plants, either in whole food form or in the form of standardized extracts and supplements, for the purpose of providing a foundation of support, both in prevention and healing. Often, I have seen these specific herbs work much faster than pharmaceuticals, without the danger of unwanted side effects. Interestingly, most drugs prescribed have roots in the plant world. By altering the chemical structure of the plant, not only does it magnify its actions (and side effects) but it also allows the drug companies to patent the medication.

Phytotherapy is much more in line with Functional Medicine, identifying and treating the underlying root cause. It's a patient-centred approach that encourages the patient and practitioner to work together inspiring the client to be their own advocate.

Conventional medicine, unfortunately, has the dangerous habit of treating symptoms alone, rarely looking at the whole canvas, let alone the individual and the picture they present. As a pharmacist, I was often shocked by the extensive overprescribing of medication.

For myself and my clients, herbs were most often the treatment of choice above all else, even the bio-identical hormones. Over the years, I became so confident with the success of Wellpoint Nutraceuticals, recognizing that if the client followed my direction, success would naturally follow. As an Integrative Practitioner, it seemed so logical to incorporate a product line into my practice to continue to guide my clients' journeys. The other choice would be to send them blindly into the 'Wild West' of a health food store or the less trustworthy internet. Other reputable products exist, however, the grade, concentration, quality control, and dosing are so variable. It's also possible to compare products per ingredient, however the manufacturing standards of practice are still an unknown, an important variable.

Incorporating herbal extracts makes these products much more powerful. Utilizing a highly concentrated herbal formula in therapeutic dosing produces long-lasting effects in conjunction with balancing not only the endocrine system, but all our body systems simultaneously. This produces such a euphoric effect with benefits that reach far beyond the intended hormone treatment for which the client is pleasantly surprised. These may include, for example, improved skin and nails, a sense of well-being, lowering of medication, less bloating, and support for other disease states.

As I started to grow my business in Integrative Medicine, my knowledge and confidence in Phytotherapy also grew. I started to learn more about the science behind the creation of pharmaceutical grade Nutraceuticals. The strength of combining multiple ingredients of concentrated herbs and herbal extracts in the products created synergy, meaning the combinations were interactive, producing a far greater benefit than the sum of each individual herb.

My next learning was proof that a multi-targeted program of dose-specific supplements produces the best and quickest results, treating the client holistically - as a whole. As you will see in the case studies, common areas of treatment with these Nutraceuticals following the template of the Saliva Hormone Test often included the following products:

Enhance for the Adrenal Gland

Life-force for Liver detox

Vita-Fem for Estrogen-Progesterone balance

Strs-ease for Cortisol

Coln-Fresh or CCLN for colon cleanse

Note: These branded supplements are distributed only through auth-orized agents/practitioners and are not available for direct sale.

Why Is the Liver the Central Component of Every Integrative Plan?

You may wonder about the connection between the liver and hormones. The liver is the central point of every program from which the targeted program can be built - like the foundation of a home. Placing the body in a state of detoxification is crucial and greatly enhances the strength of any supplement program. A healthy liver also helps to regulate the thyroid, metabolism, and the adrenal gland. For example, it metabolizes estrogen rapidly into benign metabolites. Even small excesses of estrogen can place our body in danger of unwanted illness.

Often our liver is overworked and taxed due to environmental chemicals, additives in food and drink, and an overload of medication. If our liver is taxed it can over-metabolize estrogen into a less desirable form. This metabolite could accumulate posing a serious threat to our health, especially if the client struggles with constipation and/or stress management; thus, the reasoning for a detox regimen to release the burden on the liver so it can resume its role in hormone regulation.

Similarly, by lowering cortisol the burden on our adrenal glands is lessened.

While there are similarities in the therapeutic programs created in each case study remember that the reasons and therapeutic dosages will vary for each woman due to many variables including medical history and past medication, fulfilling the goal to treat them as an individual— never a cookie-cutter integrative plan.

As you review the case studies, I am sure at least one of 'the girls' will resonate with your life experiences and may even stimulate some 'Aha' moments.

A Little More About Nutraceuticals: The Foundation of Our Success!

The nutraceutical brand I incorporated into my practice has 30-plus years' experience in the development of proprietary herbal nutraceutical formulations. All products are formulated in Canada, under the strict standards mandated by Health Canada. The manufacturing facility is GMP-certified by Health Canada among many other certifications.

Nutraceuticals and herbs are classified as natural foods. Herbs are part of our nutritional lifestyle that work synergistically with each other and proper food, allowing our body to produce remarkable cellular and organ system responses. Knowledge of these interactions and the combinations of herbal blends is what created the foundation of their proprietary formulations. By combining complementary herbs in each formulation, the chance of success is greatly increased - creating a quicker and long-lasting response. The company's belief is that natural products should be incorporated into a health regime with the guidance of a healthcare professional, specifically pharmacists due to their vast knowledge of pharmaceuticals and physiology of the human body.

Now... before you dig deep into the case studies review your hormone checklists! Come prepared and be ready for some "Aha" moments!

Case Studies: Meet the Girls

I n the following pages you'll meet actual clients I've worked with over the years who clearly illustrate the points we covered in the opening chapters. I always find it beneficial to bring together the science with examples applied to real life. It makes it meaningful and relatable.

Get out your pencil or highlighter and see what (and who) resonates with you.

CASE STUDY: COLETTE – IT'S NOT YOUR FAULT

Colette's Story: For five years Colette was treated with an oral form of HRT by her doctor. When the 5-year mark arrived, her medication was discontinued with no other form of support being offered. After multiple visits to her doctor, she threw her hands up in frustration and stopped asking for help. At the beginning of her new integrative program, she struggled with hot flashes, night sweats and insomnia. After only two weeks her energy shifted as her hot flashes began to reduce. She felt more alert and less foggy. Her bowel movements had improved with less acid reflux and bloating. She started to work on her carbohydrate restriction and her stress lowered.

Age	60
Symptoms	Hot flashes/insomnia/weight gain (50 lbs)/ night sweats/ indigestion/ bloating/ joint pain
Medical History	Diagnosed with Hypothyroidism 2013
Medication	Synthroid 0.125 (2013), HRT 2013-2018
Supplements	None to date
Areas of Concern	Weight gain stomach/ hormone imbalance/ sustainable good health/ self-esteem & energy for the grandkids
Saliva Test Results	Colette tested high for Estradiol and low for Progesterone meaning she was Estrogen Dominant. Most women assume they are very low in Estradiol, even stating "I have no Estrogen left!" This is often not the case. Her Testosterone was low, a direct indication of her struggle to maintain muscle mass. Her test also showed Adrenal Fatigue or Adrenal Dysfunction with low DHEA and high Cortisol.

TARGETED PROGRAM:

Colette's integrative program targeted the following areas:

1. Enhance balances DHEA and the Adrenal Gland. Also detoxifies the bladder and kidney. Will also improve energy levels naturally.

2. Lifeforce balances the liver and thyroid. Also good for balancing metabolism.

3. Strs-ease is an adaptogen to support stress and anxiety naturally. It also supports 'fight or flight'! Cortisol levels were high which can affect thyroid function.

4. Vita-Fem is used to balance estradiol and progesterone. It will treat current state of estrogen dominance which affects weight and thyroid. Also very effective in treating vaginal dryness and naturally rebuilding your lining, if needed. It will also improve mood swings, irritability, libido, night sweats, anxiety, and PMS symptoms.

Saliva Hormone Test Report

Patient: Collette

Salivary Hormone Results			
		Phase	Reference Range
Estradiol pmol/L	10.1	Follicular	2.8-8.8 pmol/L
		Peak*	4.5-19.1 pmol/L
		Luteal	2.8-8.2 pmol/L
		Menopausal	3.7-9.4 pmol/L
		Male	3.1-7.4 pmol/L
		*Peak = Days 11 and 12	
Testosterone pmol/L	47	Premenopausal	34-148 pmol/L
		Menopausal	34-148 pmol/L
		Male	110-513 pmol/L
Progesterone pmol/L	41	Follicular	17-321 pmol/L
		Peak *	151-829 pmol/L
		Luteal	33-452 pmol/L
		Menopausal	45-370 pmol/L
		Male	31-280 pmol/L
		*Peak = Days 18 and 20	
P/E2 Ratio	4	Follicular	10-85
		Luteal	8-80
		Menopausal	12-62
DHEA 7am-9am	296	71-640 pg/ml	
DHEA: Cortisol Ratio/10,000	1,000	358 – 2,538	

Cortisol Results	7am – 9am*	11am – 1pm*	3pm – 5pm*	10pm-12am*
Patient Result (mcg/dL)>>	0.296			
Reference Range (mcg/dL) *Based on Collection Times	0.097-0.337			
Actual Collection Time	7:39am			

CASE STUDY: HEATHER - ADRENAL FATIGUE

Heather's Story: Heather was an executive with an overwhelming commitment to her work with calls often starting at 7:00 a.m. She and her husband were very social and loved to travel. Her menstrual cycles stopped at 54 when she discontinued her birth control pills. The hot flashes were short lived, however the night sweats persisted, dramatically affecting her sleep. She often had to pull over for a quick nap on the way to work.

Her sleep improved slightly upon changing her mind-set and creating a structured nighttime routine, yet at times the night sweats were unbearable and interrupted her sleep pattern. When menopause hit, her body shape started shifting and she soon found herself 30 lbs overweight with a closet full of clothes that no longer fit properly.

Within a month of starting her integrative program her clothes were fitting better and she was down just over 10 lbs. Her energy soared and her mood swings improved. Her nights sweats started to shift, improving her sleep. While her stress levels remained high her ability to cope improved and her anxiety lessened.

Age	56
Symptoms	Brain fog, hot flashes, irritability, low sex drive, morning sluggishness, sleep disturbances, weight gain
Medical History	Long-term use of birth control pills
Medication	None
Supplements	Vitamin B, C, D, Omega, Maca, Turmeric, Magnesium
Areas of Concern	Weight gain and body fat distribution since hitting menopause. Also concerned with night sweats and mood swings. Past weight loss programs included a nutritionist and Herbal Magic.
Saliva Test Results	Heather was estrogen dominant with extremely low Progesterone which explained her irritability, mood swings, sleep disturbances

	and unwanted weight gain. She was also suffering from Adrenal Fatigue, common to women living in a stressful environment or working in a career with a demanding workload and high expectations. Her DHEA was low, limiting her body's ability to produce its own hormones and her Cortisol was extremely low (below range) affecting her sleep, weight, and morning energy.
	Her hormone panel was normal for a woman treated with long-term birth control as the drug depletes our natural hormone levels, at times throwing us into menopause early. Testosterone was also below range explaining her struggle with libido; also affected by low Progesterone.

TARGETED PROGRAM:

Heather's integrative program targeted the following areas:

1. **Adrenal Glands:** Enhance was used to balance DHEA and the Adrenal Glands offsetting the adrenal fatigue. Also used to detoxify the bladder and kidney (water retention) providing the body with a foundation of support. Balancing the adrenal glands would also improve energy levels naturally targeting morning sluggishness.

2. **Liver/Thyroid:** Lifeforce was used to detoxify the liver and thyroid. Also good for supporting and improving metabolism for weight loss.

3. **Cortisol:** Strs-ease is an adaptogen used to support our stress and anxiety naturally. It also supports our 'fight or flight.' Heather's Cortisol levels were very low which can affect thyroid function. Medium to high dosage recommended due to the level of

Cortisol which can affect the conversion of T4 to T3 (active thyroid) metabolism and weight.

4. **Estradiol/Progesterone:** Vita-Fem was used to balance estradiol and progesterone. It will treat her current state of estrogen dominance which affects weight and thyroid. Also, very effective in treating vaginal dryness and naturally rebuilding lining if needed. It will also improve mood swings, irritability, libido, night sweats, anxiety, and PMS symptoms. In Heather's case, a high dosage was recommended due to the degree of estrogen dominance.

CASE STUDY: LORRAINE – THE SECRET BLUEPRINT TO MENOPAUSE

Lorraine's Story: Lorraine was a vibrant 61-year-old woman, happily married to her second husband. She was 20 lbs or more overweight with the challenges of menopause. Her personal life was extremely stressful with extended family, leading her to eat poorly. She struggled with body image and low self-esteem due to her evolving body shape.

Her other struggle was low libido related to self-image and hormone imbalance. She also found her sleep disrupted due to repeated surges of night sweats. Within two weeks to a month her energy started to soar, and her night sweats shifted. Libido was still an issue, however, with a modification in her integrative program incorporating an herbal product called Sensuality Man, things started to work.

Age	61
Symptoms	Fatigue/insomnia, IBS (constipation, bloating, diarrhea), joint pain and stiffness, low sex drive, anxiety (situational), night sweats
Medical History	Blood Pressure, Bowel Problems (IBS), environmental allergies (Adrenal Imbalance)
Medication	Candesartan 32 mg (blood pressure), Naproxen as needed for joint pain
Supplements	Vege Greens, Protein Powder, B Complex, Vitamin C 100mg, D3 3000IU
Areas of Concern	Low libido/ weight gain/ fatigue
Saliva Test Results	To Lorraine's surprise her Estradiol and Progesterone tested high, a direct correlation to her body fat. To a degree it was like her body still thought it was cycling. In fact, if we looked at her numbers in the Luteal Phase it would look like estrogen dominance. Not having a prior reference of testing, her numbers were probably extremely high at the beginning of menopause. High numbers also meant the need to detoxify to lower hormone levels slightly. However,

her Adrenal Glands were functioning at low capacity with low DHEA and Cortisol which again was a direct relation to her high personal stress.

TARGETED PROGRAM:

Lorraine's integrative program targeted the following areas:

1. **Adrenal Glands**: Enhance was used to balance DHEA and the Adrenal Glands offsetting the adrenal fatigue. Also used to detoxify the bladder and kidney (water retention) providing the body with a foundation of support. Balancing the adrenal glands would also improve energy levels naturally, targeting morning sluggishness. Increasing Cortisol naturally would help her body to physically handle her emotional stress.

2. **Liver/Thyroid**: Lifeforce was used to detoxify the liver and thyroid. Also good for supporting and improving metabolism for weight loss. Specific to Lorraine this was an important piece to lower Estradiol and Progesterone.

3. **Cortisol**: Strs-ease is an adaptogen used to support our stress and anxiety naturally. It also supports our fight-or-flight response. Lorraine's Cortisol levels were very low which can affect thyroid function. Medium to high dosage recommended due to the level of Cortisol which can affect the conversion of T4 to T3 (active thyroid) metabolism, and weight. For Lorraine this was an important piece in her day-to-day functioning with the challenges of family dynamics.

4. **Estradiol/Progesterone**: Vita-Fem was also used to balance her high levels of estradiol and progesterone. Also, very effective in treating vaginal dryness and naturally rebuilding lining, if needed. It will also improve mood swings, irritability, libido,

night sweats, anxiety, and PMS symptoms. Overall, a powerful umbrella to targeting the emotional piece.

While Lorraine felt she handled her stress well her body embraced the natural foundation of support, improving all her symptoms and making her realize how good she could feel!

Saliva Hormone Test Report

Patient: Lorraine

Salivary Hormone Results			
		Phase	Reference Range
Estradiol pmol/L	7.4	Follicular	2.8-8.8 pmol/L
		Peak*	4.5-19.1 pmol/L
		Luteal	2.8-8.2 pmol/L
		Menopausal	3.7-9.4 pmol/L
		Male	3.1-7.4 pmol/L
		*Peak = Days 11 and 12	
Testosterone pmol/L	76	Premenopausal	34-148 pmol/L
		Menopausal	34-148 pmol/L
		Male	110-513 pmol/L
Progesterone pmol/L	276	Follicular	17-321 pmol/L
		Peak *	151-829 pmol/L
		Luteal	33-452 pmol/L
		Menopausal	45-370 pmol/L
		Male	31-280 pmol/L
		*Peak = Days 18 and 20	
P/E2 Ratio	37	Follicular	10-85
		Luteal	8-80
		Menopausal	12-62
DHEA 7am-9am	157	71-640 pg/ml	
DHEA: Cortisol Ratio/10,000	151	358 - 2,538	

Cortisol Results	7am – 9am*	11am – 1pm*	3pm – 5pm*	10pm – 12am*
Patient Result (mcg/dL)>>	1.041			
Reference Range (mcg/dL) *Based on Collection Times	0.097-0.337			
Actual Collection Time	7:38am			

CASE STUDY: ERICA – THE DANGERS OF HIGH CORTISOL

Erica's Story: Erica at 57 was very healthy. She was on no medication and had no medical history besides Menopause. She had been to multiple doctors and naturopaths with very little resolution of symptoms and areas of concern especially low libido. She didn't feel like herself and was constantly anxious. She felt extremely frustrated that none of the health care professionals she had approached could offer her the answers she was seeking. She was very happy in her marriage, yet low libido and extreme vaginal dryness was a huge issue. She often avoided sex as it was just too painful. She also struggled with frequent urinary tract infections and urinary urgency.

Age	57
Symptoms	Insomnia/ night sweats/ abdominal discomfort/ indigestion/ nausea/ constipation/ low libido/ muscle aches & pains, joint pain
Medical History	None
Medication	None
Supplements	Vitamin C, D, E, Magnesium, Collagen, Curcumin, Ashwaganda, Vitamin B Complex
Areas of Concern	Anxiety, hormonal imbalance in general, extremely low libido, vaginal dryness
Saliva Test Results	In direct correlation to her low libido, Erica tested positive for low Testosterone although this is not the only hormone related to sex drive. Her Progesterone was slightly high and her Estradiol extremely low in line with her low body fat percentage. She also struggled with Adrenal Dysfunction, not uncommon at her age, with high DHEA and high Cortisol. She often felt wired yet tired and anxious, like her body was running on high.

TARGETED PROGRAM:

Erica's integrative program targeted the following areas:

1. **Adrenal Glands**: Enhance was used to balance DHEA and the Adrenal Glands offsetting the Adrenal Dysfunction. Also used to detoxify the bladder and kidney (water retention), providing the body with a foundation of support. Balancing the adrenal glands would also improve energy levels naturally and provide her body with the tools to naturally produce Estradiol to overcome vaginal dryness.

2. **Liver/Thyroid**: Lifeforce was used to detoxify the liver and thyroid providing the bodies organs with a foundation of support.

3. **Cortisol & Testosterone**: Sensuality Man is an adaptogen used to support our stress and anxiety naturally plus provide the body with the tools to increases its own testosterone levels naturally. It also supports our fight or flight. Erica's Cortisol levels were very high which can affect thyroid function. Medium to high dosage recommended due to the level of Cortisol which can affect the conversion of T4 to T3 (active thyroid). Her Testosterone was also low affecting her sex drive along with vaginal dryness.

4. **Estradiol/Progesterone**: Vita-Fem was used to balance estradiol and progesterone. Very effective in treating vaginal dryness and naturally re-building lining instead of using medicinal Vagifem which could negatively affect her partner's Estradiol. It will also improve mood swings, irritability, libido, night sweats, anxiety, and PMS symptoms.

Saliva Hormone Test Report

Patient: Erica

Salivary Hormone Results			
		Phase	Reference Range
Estradiol pmol/L	2.7	Follicular	2.8-8.8 pmol/L
		Peak*	4.5-19.1 pmol/L
		Luteal	2.8-8.2 pmol/L
		Menopausal	3.7-9.4 pmol/L
		Male	3.1-7.4 pmol/L
		*Peak = Days 11 and 12	
Testosterone pmol/L	47	Premenopausal	34-148 pmol/L
		Menopausal	34-148 pmol/L
		Male	110-513 pmol/L
Progesterone pmol/L	347	Follicular	17-321 pmol/L
		Peak *	151-829 pmol/L
		Luteal	33-452 pmol/L
		Menopausal	45-370 pmol/L
		Male	31-280 pmol/L
		*Peak = Days 18 and 20	
P/E2 Ratio	129	Follicular	10-85
		Luteal	8-80
		Menopausal	12-62
DHEA 7am-9am	585	71-640 pg/ml	
DHEA: Cortisol Ratio/10,000	1,548	358 – 2,538	

Cortisol Results	7am – 9am*	11am – 1pm*	3pm – 5pm*	10pm–12am*
Patient Result (mcg/dL)>>	0.378			
Reference Range (mcg/dL) *Based on Collection Times	0.097-0.337			
Actual Collection Time	7:27am			

CASE STUDY: VERONICA - RELEASING HORMONAL WEIGHT

Veronica's Story: When I met Veronica, she had a weight loss goal of 30 to 50 lbs. She told me that she had never been slim however, in the past, could always lose weight with small diet modifications and increased physical activity. For the last 2-3 years she felt her body was gaining weight differently and for the first time in her life her self-image didn't match the person in the mirror. Emotionally the shift in body weight made her feel old and unattractive. Her physical health was being impacted with a slight increase in blood pressure and challenges with mobility and joint stiffness. With a hysterectomy at 40, she recognized there could also be a hormonal component. Her intention was to be healthy, feel healthy and feel good about her self-image. At the end of her program, she surpassed her goal losing 75 lbs reaching her pre-university weight!

Age	55
Symptoms	Insomnia/ night sweats/ fatigue/ excessive weight gain
Medical History	MS diagnosis 2007
Medication	None
Supplements	Vitamin D 1000 IU 3x daily
Areas of Concern	Weight loss for better health and to increase mobility
Saliva Test Results	Her saliva panel showed very low levels of all her hormones except the Cortisol which tested very high. Low levels were a result of her hysterectomy which forced her body into surgical menopause. With no support her hormone levels became very depleted and had no resource from her Adrenal Gland to chronologically re-build itself. Her body was in a state of Adrenal Fatigue. She was experiencing high fatigue and lack of motivation. High Cortisol also affected her Thyroid and metabolism making it challenging to release weight.

TARGETED PROGRAM:

Veronica's integrative program targeted the following areas:

1. **Adrenal Glands:** Enhance was used to balance DHEA and the Adrenal Glands offsetting her adrenal fatigue. Also used to detoxify the bladder and kidney (water retention) providing the body with a foundation of support and improved circulation to treat her fluctuations in blood pressure. Balancing the adrenal glands would also improve energy levels naturally targeting morning sluggishness and restoring her body's natural ability to provide the building blocks to improve hormone levels such as Estradiol and Progesterone chronologically.

2. **Liver/Thyroid:** Lifeforce was used to detoxify the liver and balance thyroid. Also good for supporting and improving metabolism to enhance her weight loss.

3. **Cortisol:** Strs-ease is an adaptogen used to support stress and anxiety naturally. It also supports fight or flight. Veronica's Cortisol levels were very high which can affect thyroid function. Medium to high dosage was recommended due to the level of Cortisol which has a direct affect on the conversion of T4 to T3 (active thyroid) metabolism and weight.

4. **Estradiol/Progesterone:** Vita-Fem was used to balance estradiol and progesterone. Veronica's levels were very low due to the implications of her hysterectomy and lack of treatment thereafter. Also, very effective in treating vaginal dryness and naturally re-building lining, if needed, in place of prescription Vagifem. While Veronica did not exhibit excessive symptoms of mood swings, irritability, low libido, night sweats, anxiety, or PMS, the treatment did improve her mind-set and overall sense of well-being!

Saliva Hormone Test Report

Patient: Veronica

Salivary Hormone Results			
		Phase	Reference Range
Estradiol pmol/L	3.9	Follicular	2.8-8.8 pmol/L
		Peak*	4.5-19.1 pmol/L
		Luteal	2.8-8.2 pmol/L
		Menopausal	3.7-9.4 pmol/L
		Male	3.1-7.4 pmol/L
		*Peak = Days 11 and 12	
Testosterone pmol/L	<30	Premenopausal	34-148 pmol/L
		Menopausal	34-148 pmol/L
		Male	110-513 pmol/L
Progesterone pmol/L	148	Follicular	17-321 pmol/L
		Peak *	151-829 pmol/L
		Luteal	33-452 pmol/L
		Menopausal	45-370 pmol/L
		Male	31-280 pmol/L
		*Peak = Days 18 and 20	
P/E2 Ratio	38	Follicular	10-85
		Luteal	8-80
		Menopausal	12-62
DHEA 7am-9am	189	71-640 pg/ml	
DHEA: Cortisol Ratio/10,000	524	358 – 2,538	

Cortisol Results	7am – 9am*	11am – 1pm*	3pm – 5pm*	10pm-12am*
Patient Result (mcg/dL)>>	0.361			
Reference Range (mcg/dL) *Based on Collection Times	0.097-0.337			
Actual Collection Time	7:43am			

CASE STUDY: TAYLORE - ESTROGEN DOMINANCE

Taylore's Story: At 58 years old Taylore had never experienced any health issues and was on zero medication. Her nutrition was balanced, her body weight and shape were aligned, and she worked out 3 to 5 times a week. As she would say she drank lots of water and ate lots of kale! Menopause however had its challenges. Like many women, even though she felt prepared, she really had no expectation of how that journey would present itself. As her cycles slowed, she started to experience a multitude of symptoms the worst of which was very heavy, debilitating cycles that took over her life. Not wanting to embrace the medication her doctor kindly recommended she decided her first step was to complete a Saliva Hormone Test.

Age	58
Symptoms	Mild mood swings and irritability, extremely heavy cycles, slight depression, low sex drive
Medical History	Nothing significant to report except four healthy children! Family history of breast cancer.
Medication	Zero
Supplements	Extensive after years of working in Integrative Medicine
Areas of Concern	Heavy menstrual periods
Saliva Test Results	Surprisingly Taylore's test results showed high Estradiol even though she had low body fat. A testimony to the benefit of testing as most women assume their Estradiol is low and may gravitate towards the wrong supplementation. In fact, she was in a state of Estrogen Dominance, a risk factor due to the family history of breast cancer. The degree of Estrogen Dominance was high as her Progesterone was very low explaining the heavy menstrual cycles. Her adrenal glands were in balance. In fact, her Cortisol was right in the middle of normal. Another surprise due to the stress of her environment.

TARGETED PROGRAM:

Taylore's integrative program targeted the following areas:

1. **Adrenal Glands:** Enhance was used to support DHEA and the Adrenal Glands for maintenance. Also used to detoxify the bladder and kidney (water retention) providing the body with a foundation of support. A very important step used to lower and eliminate high hormone levels.

2. **Liver/Thyroid:** Lifeforce was used to detoxify the liver and thyroid. In addition, in combination with the Colon cleanse targeting the elimination of high hormone levels.

3. **Colon Cleanse:** Used to provide the full support of cleansing and eliminating fat soluble hormone levels.

4. **Estradiol/Progesterone:** Vita-Fem was used at a low dosage to balance estradiol and progesterone. It will treat her current state of estrogen dominance which affects heavy cycles and thyroid. It will also improve mood swings, irritability, libido, night sweats, anxiety, and PMS symptoms. In Taylore's case, a low dosage was recommended as the priority was to cleanse and lower Estradiol.

Saliva Hormone Test Report

Patient: Taylore

Salivary Hormone Results			
		Phase	Reference Range
Estradiol pmol/L	7.8	Follicular	2.8-8.8 pmol/L
		Peak*	4.5-19.1 pmol/L
		Luteal	2.8-8.2 pmol/L
		Menopausal	3.7-9.4 pmol/L
		Male	3.1-7.4 pmol/L
		*Peak = Days 11 and 12	
Testosterone pmol/L	<30	Premenopausal	34-148 pmol/L
		Menopausal	34-148 pmol/L
		Male	110-513 pmol/L
Progesterone pmol/L	<16	Follicular	17-321 pmol/L
		Peak *	151-829 pmol/L
		Luteal	33-452 pmol/L
		Menopausal	45-370 pmol/L
		Male	31-280 pmol/L
		*Peak = Days 18 and 20	
P/E2 Ratio	2	Follicular	10-85
		Luteal	8-80
		Menopausal	12-62
DHEA 7am-9am	406	71-640 pg/ml	
DHEA: Cortisol Ratio/10,000	1,933	358 – 2,538	

Cortisol Results	7am – 9am*	11am-1pm*	3pm – 5pm*	10pm-12am*
Patient Result (mcg/dL)>>	0.210			
Reference Range (mcg/dL) *Based on Collection Times	0.097-0.337			
Actual Collection Time	7:05am			

CASE STUDY: SANDRA – COMMITTING TO SELF-CARE

Sandra's Story: Like many women Sandra was all consumed with work and the responsibilities at home. Her health was deeply challenged, yet she refused to put herself first, even after her diagnosis of breast cancer. Her family history of breast and ovarian cancer was extensive and heartbreaking. Sadly, her maternal ancestors carried the BRCA1 mutation. By 2014, Sandra made a wise decision to have an oophorectomy. By then her mom had died of ovarian cancer, multiple aunts of breast cancer and her sister was struggling with both ovarian and breast cancer.

Surgical menopause hit hard with multiple symptoms from intense hot flashes to weight gain. Surprisingly her doctors put her on HRT, not a best choice with her history, yet she felt euphoric. After her diagnosis of breast cancer in 2019 the carpet was pulled out from under her, HRT was discontinued, and her symptoms came back with a vengeance. With multiple drug therapies her weight shifted again dramatically. Her body was so off balance she became a sugar and caffeine addict. She literally felt like "she was going to jump out of her own skin."

Her goal was to work toward decreasing the dosages of medication and shifting towards integrative medicine. Within a month of treatment, her hot flashes started to subside to a degree (yet not perfect!) and her sleep improved. Her biggest challenge, however, was living in a troubled marriage and a non-supportive toxic environment.

Age	50
Symptoms	Fatigue, anxiety, depression, insomnia, hot flashes, night sweats, excessive weight gain, low libido
Medical History	Breast Cancer- double mastectomy 2019, heart disease (valve replacement), Oophorectomy 2018

Medication	Citalopram 20mg (depression), Gabapentin 600-900mg (nerve damage/hot flashes), Aspirin 80mg, Zoplicone as needed (sleeping pill)
Supplements	Vitamin D 4000 IU, Magnesium 600mg daily, CBD oil as needed
Areas of Concern	Sleep and all her symptoms associated with surgical menopause
Saliva Test Results	Surprisingly her estrogen came back low, a gift with her history of breast cancer. Her Progesterone, however, was high, the reverse of Heather yet creating a similar picture of irritability, mood swings, sleep disturbances and unwanted weight. In addition, her Testosterone tested extremely low. In combination with her high Progesterone, it provided an explanation for her low, almost non-existent sex drive. Like many women her age she struggled with Adrenal Fatigue. Her DHEA was slightly past the middle range for menopause and her Cortisol tested twice above the highest range. This certainly explained her extreme discomfort, edginess, and unsettledness - like she was "going out of her mind." Her body was so wired, it explained her struggle to settle her mind and body for a peaceful night of sleep.

TARGETED PROGRAM:

Sandra's integrative program targeted the following areas:

1. **Adrenal Glands:** Enhance was used to balance DHEA and the Adrenal Glands offsetting the adrenal fatigue. Also used to detoxify the bladder and kidney (water retention) providing the body with a foundation of support. Balancing the adrenal glands would also improve energy levels providing her body with the natural building tools to build her hormone levels chronologically.

2. **Liver/Thyroid**: Lifeforce was used to detoxify the liver and thyroid. Also good for supporting and improving metabolism for weight loss. In Sandra's case it was important to support the liver to off-set the side effect of all the medication and their metabolites circulating in her system.

3. **Cortisol**: Strs-ease is an adaptogen used to support our stress and anxiety naturally. It also supports our fight or flight. Sandra's Cortisol levels were extremely high as expected with her physical and emotional stress, which can affect thyroid function. High dosages recommended due to the level of Cortisol which can affect the conversion of T4 to T3 (active thyroid) metabolism and weight plus anxiety.

4. **Estradiol/Progesterone**: Vita-Fem was used to balance estradiol and progesterone. It will treat her estradiol-progesterone axis, partners that struggle work together (a reason why estrogen should never be used alone!). This imbalance dramatically affects weight and thyroid. Also, very effective in treating vaginal dryness and naturally re-building lining if needed. It will also improve mood swings, irritability, libido, night sweats, anxiety, and PMS symptoms. In Sandra's case a regular dosage was recommended recognizing the Progesterone is a very emotional hormone. In her case, however, Cortisol was the top priority.

Saliva Hormone Test Report

Patient: Sandra

Salivary Hormone Results			
		Phase	Reference Range
Estradiol pmol/L	4.5	Follicular	2.8-8.8 pmol/L
		Peak*	4.5-19.1 pmol/L
		Luteal	2.8-8.2 pmol/L
		Menopausal	3.7-9.4 pmol/L
		Male	3.1-7.4 pmol/L
		*Peak = Days 11 and 12	
Testosterone pmol/L	<30	Premenopausal	34-148 pmol/L
		Menopausal	34-148 pmol/L
		Male	110-513 pmol/L
Progesterone pmol/L	253	Follicular	17-321 pmol/L
		Peak *	151-829 pmol/L
		Luteal	33-452 pmol/L
		Menopausal	45-370 pmol/L
		Male	31-280 pmol/L
		*Peak = Days 18 and 20	
P/E2 Ratio	56	Follicular	10-85
		Luteal	8-80
		Menopausal	12-62
DHEA 7am-9am	367	71-640 pg/ml	
DHEA: Cortisol Ratio/10,000	495	358 – 2,538	

Cortisol Results	7am – 9am*	11am – 1pm*	3pm – 5pm*	10pm-12am*
Patient Result (mcg/dL)>>	0.741			
Reference Range (mcg/dL) *Based on Collection Times	0.097-0.337			
Actual Collection Time	7:18am			

Your Next Steps:
How to Take Control Back

O nce your chemistry is established by the saliva hormone test, it is married with the health profile assessment which lists symptoms, medical history (family and personal), current and past medication, supplements, and areas of concern. By combining both, the client is given a whole integrative approach and a solid foundation to supporting not only their hormonal health but all aspects of their health including any current disease states. With an integrative approach the benefits are endless!

While bio-identical hormones may still be on the table for low hormone levels, the best approach is to combine that with a detoxification program for kidney/bladder, liver, and colon. This will provide a very solid foundation to continuously bring the body in balance and avoid the unwanted side effects of medication. No matter which treatment option is best suited to the client, detoxification creates the infrastructure for our body systems, the building blocks.

I always explain to clients that our best option is to put "all the cards on the table at once" and multi-target at least four areas for best resolution of symptoms and quickest results. Low hormone levels can be targeted with BHRT or herbal supplements; high hormone levels need to be targeted with herbs and detoxification. Also bear in mind that body fat will store excess hormones, so weight release is always a consideration in bringing hormones in line. In fact, if a woman is obese there is a high risk of storing hormones if either HRT or BHRT is used.

Releasing weight also provides the client with another important pillar of their customized journey - lifestyle modification, renewed self-esteem, confidence and in many cases disease prevention. Again, a whole integrative approach including the thyroid and the entire hormone cascade.

One of women's frustrations in attempting to seek the support of their physician (that I have seen again and again) is the thyroid is often treated alone or dismissed entirely. Blood work does not always accurately tell the story or match the client's symptoms. Our best assumption is that the thyroid is off balance as the other hormones are changing. By providing the foundational support of herbs the client can naturally target their thyroid as well with or without medication. Pharmaceuticals weaken the thyroid over time as we've discussed in more detail in an earlier chapter.

With any treatment option our best window of opportunity for full resolution is a solid three months. With Bio-Identical Hormone Replacement Therapy (BHRT) it is best to ride out the same dosages for two months before considering any changes. Herbs are much easier to adjust along the way. Plus, clients often see faster results on the herbs if multi-targeted at appropriate therapeutic dosages. I am very confident in the outcome, and my clients are often happily surprised. At the 3-month window, herbal dosages can often be slowly decreased to test the clients baseline ability to sustain the euphoric results of the herbs.

So, What Does a Therapeutic Herbal Plan Look Like?

Multitargeting with herbs and the foundation of detoxification is best achieved by utilizing four supplements to target multiple areas with products and dosages based on the health assessment, married with the saliva hormone results. A Therapeutic Plan often means using a customized combination of:

    a. a supplement to balance estradiol and progesterone

    b. a supplement to balance the adrenal gland and DHEA

    c. a supplement to balance liver and thyroid in combination

    d. a supplement to balance Cortisol, and/or

    e. a supplement to balance low testosterone and low libido.

Dosages will vary between clients contingent on the degree of their symptoms and their medical history. For example: a hysterectomy, thyroid disease, long term use of birth control or HRT. I feel assertive programs are best as often women have been in the 'pit' of menopause for years, frustrated and disheartened.

Understand that BHRT may leave you feeling euphoric in the beginning, thinking you've found the answer! But the results will start tapering off. With BHRT alone, client dosages will often have to be increased as women will build up a tolerance to the medication like many prescribed medications.

If herbs are not incorporated, some areas of imbalance will often be left untreated. By adding complementary herbal support to the BHRT, you are increasing your chances of a long-term, full range of success. *However, understand that from my perspective an integrative plan of herbs alone is always our best go-to, totally natural with absolutely no risk of side effects.*

#1: STRESS MANANAGEMENT: THE HOPE OF BALANCING CORTISOL

Stressful events are a fact of life and often not within our control. And you may not be able to change your current situation. However, you can take steps to manage the impact these events have on you.

You can learn to identify what causes your stress and how to take care of yourself physically, emotionally, and spiritually in the face of these stressful circumstances.

Your stress management strategies should include:

➢ Eating a healthy diet, getting regular exercise, and getting plenty of sleep

➢ Creating a very structured morning routine

➢ Practicing relaxation techniques such as yoga, deep breathing, massage, or meditation

➢ Keeping a journal and writing about your thoughts or what you're grateful for in your daily life

➢ Taking time for hobbies, such as reading, listening to music, or taking lessons to learn something new

➢ Fostering healthy friendships and relationships with friends and family

➢ Having a sense of humour and finding ways to include humour and laughter in your life

➢ Volunteering in your community

➢ Organizing and prioritizing what you need to accomplish at home and work and removing tasks that aren't necessary

➢ Seeking professional counseling if required to help you develop specific coping strategies to manage stress

➢ Avoiding unhealthy stimulants to manage your stress that don't serve you, such as using alcohol, tobacco, overprescribed prescription drugs or excess sugar.

The rewards for learning to manage stress are far-reaching and limitless, including:

➢ peace of mind and tranquility,

➢ less anxiety and improved sleep,

➢ a better quality and enjoyment of life,

➢ improvement and transition to better health,

➢ better self-control, focus, and clarity, and

➢ better relationships

…. leading to a longer, healthier life! A journey of joy and gratitude.

Think back to the earlier chapters and checklists where we explored stress hormones. One of our top five hormones to balance is Cortisol. Its role in a successful integrative plan is crucial. Cortisol directly affects thyroid, metabolism, and your ability to release unwanted weight (especially the 'menopause muffin').

Which brings us to the next consideration for your integrative plan and overall health... weight release!

#2: Why Weight and Body Image Are Always Our Focus!

Why do women focus on the release of unwanted weight as part of the hormone testing and management plan? Well, #1 we get tired of fighting the muffin top and recognize our body starts to gain weight differently during menopause. We look back at pictures in despair, too often afraid to look in the mirror, frustrated with how our clothes fit.

As our weight is tied to our health in so many ways, having our weight under control often means better outcomes for many health conditions. It also means a sense of self control, self-confidence, a renewed energy and commitment to self-care, and general wellbeing.

Think about what it feels like when your clothes fit comfortably, and how your focus and energy soars along with renewed self-esteem! It's an amazing feeling! Yet it can be an uphill battle with many challenges and pieces to the puzzle. However, as you saw with Veronica the outcome is always worth embracing change, reaching our goals & sustaining a reasonable lifestyle!! Now let's review.....

So, Let's Review What We've Done...

We've discussed what menopause is. That it is not a disease but a transition and journey, the final chapter. We've defined what hormones do for us and why our body struggles to overcome symptoms of imbalance. We've reviewed the symptoms you can experience when your hormones are out of balance with a little a bit of science. I've introduced you to a number of clients, "The Girls" (there are hundreds) who have experienced real results, in the hope you can relate to at least a few of them, bringing clarity and empathy to your journey. Perhaps even a few 'A-Ha!' moments.

I've provided several resources to assist you to understand that the changes happening to your body (inside and out) are part of a natural process, not a disease state and, most importantly, that it's not your fault you didn't have ALL the answers in the beginning.

Now it's time for you to embrace this knowledge, clarify what your next steps are and take charge. Develop an accountability plan with small steps in the beginning and goal setting. Remember it's up to us to initiate change!

My advice is to start with a totally objective test that defines what's happening within your body now, and that allows you to develop a truly personal blueprint for the next steps based on your unique chemistry. A blueprint to support your body physically and emotionally as you start your new journey. Begin now to create a limitless life by painting your perception with a positive mindset and gratitude... aligned with the best version of your true self.

The Last Step...
Manifesting Gratitude and
Paving the Way for the Future

Always begin your gratitude session by thinking of your day, focusing on the big and small events. Focus on the gifts you experienced today (in the beginning you may need to search a bit to recognize moments and gestures). Acknowledge the challenges as gifts of learning to make you more resilient and stronger (such as managing a disagreement with intelligence not emotion).

Setting the practice of journaling should always be scheduled into our day. Being grateful in the beginning does not always come naturally. The act of writing will consolidate your thoughts into your memory and subconscious mind, like the hard drive on your computer. It will also start to manifest your future and create the events you so desire. Your thoughts will co-create your future.

Reflection is the unhurried consideration of an event with the threads of spirituality. Consider the following questions:

1. What was the lesson?

2. What made this a positive event?

3. What was the challenge?

4. What did I have to overcome?

5. How does it make me feel deep in my heart?

6. How will this event enrich my life?

Individuals who practice gratitude and manifestation have the tendency to....

➤ Enjoy a sense of contentment (and realize their future goals)

➤ Combat adversity with grace

➤ Feel more energized and at peace

➤ Sleep more contently

➤ Have lower levels of Cortisol (hence a stronger immune system)

➤ Treat the world with kindness and compassion

Remember: your sub-conscious mind doesn't know the difference between the present and the future. Manifesting our future through thought alone creates the event as though it has already occurred. *Ask for what you want!*

START PAVING THE WAY FOR YOUR FUTURE…YOUR TURNING POINT

Describe what your ideal life would be like one year from now:

_____

_____

_____

_____

What needs to change in order to achieve your ideal life?

_____

_____

_____

_____

Are you ready to make those changes?

_____

_____

_____

_____

Do you know how to make those changes?

_____

_____

_____

_____

What resources can you draw on to make these changes?

_____

_____

_____

_____

I'd like to suggest that reading this book was one of your resources!

Conclusion

Managing day-to-day life often leaves women unprepared for menopause, too depleted to take on its unpredictable adventures; however, there is a clear path to resolving our worst menopausal symptoms. A path that will allow us to find peace and tranquility, hope and renewed self-esteem.

My message to women is to not give up. We do not have to just accept all these changes as part of aging. It is possible to find the true answers and solutions you so desperately seek, specific to your journey and desired outcome. It's just that the solutions must be customized to you!

So, start at the beginning, and don't make any assumptions. The test results always speak for themselves with validation and accuracy. Think of menopause as a journey, and the Saliva Hormone Test as the map, the tool directing you towards your personalized destination and future goals of SELF-CARE, HEALTH and HAPPINESS!

Congratulations on starting your new journey. For finally making yourself a priority. Now is your time! Begin today to create the life you want!

About the Author

Kelly Nolan is a Pharmacist, Integrative Practitioner, and mother of 4 healthy children. For over 30 plus years she has mentored women's passage thru peri-menopause & menopause by sharing her expertise, and teaching women to put their self-care at the forefront in order to be the care giver to those around them. Transitioning to Integrative Medicine with the foundation of a pharmacist & scientist, she has been able to educate her clients on the value of blending herbs with traditional medicine, and supporting all aspects of their health with high-grade natural supplements in combination with a healthy lifestyle & stress management. She has become a leader in her field, an expert in the healing arts of women's health.

What's Next On
Your Menopause Journey?

The end of this book marks the beginning of your new journey. Start by lining up all the tools you need!

Be committed & accountable to your own self-care! Get access to all these beautiful tools & resources to fill your Menopause Kit accessible on-line at www.hormonetesting.ca.

Avita Hormone Balancing Package:

Take charge and "Restore Your Life" with the Saliva Hormone Test, the road map to navigating your menopause journey with tailored solutions specific to your chemistry. The most important tool in your "Menopause Kit!"

The Avita Hormone Balancing Workbook:

Helpful resources to provide a teaching platform to guide your journey. Worksheets & tools to document your current symptoms and track your progress. Resources create awareness and commitment to finding your true answers & being accountable to change.

The Menopause Quiz:

If you are experiencing symptoms such as weight gain, night sweats, mood swings, insomnia and more its time to take control back. This Success

Formula Worksheet is an important step to understanding how your hormones are impacting your health, relationships, and self-image. Getting your score will define your next steps and provide clarity. Your quiz results will be sent directly to Kelly Nolan for evaluation.

Private Facebook Group: "Restore Your Life":

Join our safe community of "like -minded women" to share your stories and be heard by asking for advice & direction. Remember all these women "have walked in your shoes". Embrace their wisdom, support and life experiences that could enhance your journey.

Join our Private Facebook Group
Facebook.com/groups/430263684686587

Social Media Links

Facebook.com/AvitaRestorativeHealth

LinkedIn.com/in/Kelly-Nolan-1993132b/

Instagram.com/KellyNolanAvita/

YouTube.com/channel/UCbkUa5fm3QH_HEk7OeOWvjw

Made in the USA
Middlctown, DE
24 February 2023

25362284R00104